Recent Results in Cancer Research

Fortschritte der Krebsforschung

Progrès dans les recherches sur le cancer

7

W0227875

Edited by

V. G. Allfrey, New York · M. Allgöwer, Chur · K. H. Bauer, Heidelberg · I. Berenblum, Rehovoth · F. Bergel, Jersey/C. I. · J. Bernard, Paris · W. Bernhard, Villejuif N. N. Blokhin, Moskva · H. E. Bock, Tübingen · P. Bucalossi, Milano · A. V. Chaklin, Moskva · M. Chorazy, Gliwice · G. J. Cunningham, London · W. Dameshek, Boston M. Dargent, Lyon · G. Della Porta, Milano · P. Denoix, Villejuif · R. Dulbecco, San Diego · H. Eagle, New York · R. Eker, Oslo · P. Grabar, Paris · H. Hamperl, Bonn R. J. C. Harris, London · E. Hecker, Heidelberg · R. Herbeuval, Nancy · J. Higginson, Lyon · W. C. Hueper, Bethesda · H. Isliker, Lausanne · D. A. Karnofsky, New York · J. Kieler, København · G. Klein, Stockholm · H. Koprowski, Philadelphia · L. G. Koss, New York · G. Martz, Zürich · G. Mathé, Paris · O. Mühlbock, Amsterdam · G. T. Pack, New York · V. R. Potter, Madison · A. B. Sabin, Cincinnati · L. Sachs, Rehovoth · E. A. Saxén, Helsinki · W. Szybalski, Madison H. Tagnon, Bruxelles · R. M. Taylor, Toronto · A. Tissières, Genève · E. Uehlinger, Zürich · R. W. Wissler, Chicago · T. Yoshida, Tokyo · L.A. Zilber, Moskva

Editor in chief
P. Rentchnick, Genève

Springer-Verlag · New York, Inc. 1966

Multiple Primary Malignant Neoplasms

Their Incidence and Significance

Charles G. Moertel

With 19 Figures

Springer-Verlag New York Inc. 1966

Charles G. Moertel, M.D., M.S. in Medicine, Consultant, Section of Medicine and Section of Clinical Oncology, Mayo Clinic

Assistant Professor of Medicine, Mayo Graduate School of Medicine (University of Minnesota)

Sponsored by the Swiss League against Cancer

Acknowledgment

The author acknowledges with gratitude the collaboration of the following investigators in portions of this work: HOWARD A. ANDERSEN, M. D.; ARCHIE H. BAGGENSTOSS, M. D.; J. ARNOLD BARGEN, M. D.; MALCOLM B. DOCKERTY, M. D.; EDWARD L. FOSS, M. D.; ALBERT B. HAGEDORN, M. D.; KEITH E. HOLLEY, M. D.; EDWARD H. SOULE, M. D.

In addition, he wishes to extend credit to the following publishers for their kind permission to use material published previously in the journals indicated: The Williams & Wilkins Company (*Gastroenterology*); Grune & Stratton, Inc. (*Blood*); J. B. Lippincott Company (*Annals of Surgery, Cancer*); The American College of Surgeons (*Surgery, Gynecology & Obstetrics*); and the American College of Chest Physicians (*Diseases of the Chest*).

ISBN 978-3-642-87567-0   ISBN 978-3-642-87565-6 (eBook)
DOI 10.1007/978-3-642-87565-6

Table of Contents

A. Introduction and Presentation of Data   1

   1. Criteria for Diagnosis   2

   2. Classification   3

   3. Selection of Cases for Our Study   4

   4. Observations   4

   5. Rate of Occurrence   6

   6. Report of Cases   8

   Summary 19

   References 20

B. Multiple Primary Malignant Neoplasms of Different Tissues or Organs 21

   1. Introductory Comments 21
      Reference 22

   2. Occurrence of Multiple Cancers within the Same or Related Organ Systems . . 22
      a) Multiple Cancers Involving the Female Genitalia and Breasts 22
      b) Coexistence of Epithelial Carcinoma of the Bladder and Adenocarcinoma of
         the Prostate 25

      References 25

   3. Second Primary Cancers Induced by Treatment of an Initial Malignant Neoplasm 25
      a) Therapeutic Ionizing Radiation 26
      b) The Stewart-Treves Syndrome 27
      c) Carcinoma of the Male Breast Developing during Estrogen Therapy for Carci-
         noma of the Prostate 28

      References 29

   4. Hereditary Influences in Patients with Multiple Primary Malignant Neoplasms . 30

      References 32

   5. Blood Groups and Multiple Primary Malignant Neoplasms 32

      References 34

   6. Leukemia or Lymphoma and Coexistent Primary Malignant Neoplasms 34
      a) Cases Reported in the Literature 37
      b) Selection of Our Cases for Study 40
      c) Leukemia Plus Malignant Lesions 41
      d) Lymphoma Plus another Malignant Lesion 43
      e) Coexistence of Kaposi's Sarcoma and Leukemia or Lymphoma 44

f) Coexistence of Epitheliomas of the Skin and Chronic Lymphatic Leukemia . 47
g) Cancer and Acute Leukemias: Effects of Radiation 48
h) Incidence 49
i) Comment 50

Summary 50

References 50

7. Carcinoid Tumors of the Small Intestine and Second Primary Cancers 57

References 59

8. The Coexistence of Primary Lung Cancer and Other Primary Malignant Neoplasms 59
a) Selection of Cases 60
b) Observations 60
c) Comment 61

Summary 62

References 63

C. Multiple Primary Malignant Neoplasms of Multicentric Origin 63

1. Introductory Comments 63

References 63

2. Multicentric Epitheliomas of the Skin 64

References 64

3. Multicentric Carcinomas of the Oral Cavity 64
a) Selection of Cases 65
b) Observations 65
c) Comment 67
Summary 67

References 67

4. Multicentric Epitheliomas of the Lips 67

References 68

5. Multicentric Epitheliomas Involving the Larynx, Pharynx, and Esophagus . . 68

Reference 69

6. Multicentric Adenocarcinomas of the Stomach 69
a) Present Study 69
b) Results 70
c) Comment 74

References 75

7. Multicentric Carcinoid Tumors 75

References 76

8. Multicentric Adenocarcinomas of the Colon and Rectum 76
a) Selection of Cases 77
b) Results 78
c) Comment 86
Summary 87

References 87

9. Multicentric Epitheliomas of the Urinary Tract 88

a) Multicentric Tumors of the Bladder 89
b) Multicentric Lesions Associated with Neoplasms of the Renal Pelvis . . . 90

References 90

10. Multicentric Carcinomas of the Cervix, Vagina, Vulva, and Anus 91

Reference 91

11. Bilateral Carcinomas of the Breast 91
a) Criteria for the Diagnosis of Independent Cancer in the Second Breast . . 92
b) Observations 93
c) Unsimultaneous (Nonsynchronous) Cancer in the Second Breast 93
d) Simultaneous (Synchronous) Cancer in the Second Breast 95
e) Independent Cancers of the Second Breast in Association with Other Primary
    Malignant Neoplasms 97
f) Comment 97
g) The Problem of Prophylactic Simple Mastectomy of the Second Breast . . 97
Summary 99

References 100

12. Bilateral Testicular Cancers 100

References 101

13. Bilateral Ovarian Carcinomas 101

References 102

14. Multicentric Bronchial Carcinomas 102

References 102

15. Multicentric Carcinomas of Parenchymatous Organs 103
a) Multicentric Carcinomas of the Kidney 103
b) Multicentric Carcinomas of the Thyroid and Pancreas 103
c) Multicentric Hepatomas 103

Reference 103

16. Multicentric Gliomas of the Central Nervous System 103

References 104

17. Multicentric Malignant Neoplasms of the Reticuloendothelial System 104

Reference 104

18. The Case for Multicentricity of Origin of Malignant Neoplasms 104

References 106

Summary 107

A. Introduction and Presentation of Data

... so ist wohl auch die Annahme nicht auszuschließen, daß bei einem Individuum sich zweimal im Leben Carcinom entwickeln kann, wenn das erste Mal radikale Heilung durch die Operation erzielt worden war. (BILLROTH)

Although a few poorly documented reports of cases of multiple primary malignant neoplasms may be found in the earlier literature, the real foundation and stimulus for study of this interesting phenomenon was provided by BILLROTH in 1889, when he documented several cases of more than one independent cancer developing in the same patient.

The spark of interest generated by BILLROTH was kept alive only by a few isolated case reports in the later years of the nineteenth century, and the patient with multiple cancers was viewed with the same detached curiosity by the medical profession as the freaks exploited by P. T. BARNUM were being viewed by the laity. Throughout this century, however, the frequency of reports of multiple primary malignant tumors has increased so steadily that they have now become a commonplace and significant problem. By 1932 WARREN and GATES were able to collect 1,259 cases from the world literature. Over the last 3 decades, the number of reported cases has increased in an almost exponential fashion. A careful, but undoubtedly incomplete, compilation of the cases reported to the time of this writing revealed more than 20,000 cases of multiple primary malignant neoplasms documented by several hundred authors whose publications range in size from innumerable single case reports to the study by MERSHEIMER and associates of 4,230 cases.

Not only has the absolute number of cases reported increased in recent years, but the frequency of occurrence of this phenomenon has seemed to increase also. Typical of the general trend in the literature are two reports by WARREN and his associates. Using autopsy cases they found that 3.7% of all patients with malignant neoplasms seen from 1926 through 1931 had multiple primary lesions; whereas 6.8% of the patients with malignant tumors seen from 1932 through 1943 had multiple primary cancers. A similar trend is seen in reports of surgical cases. HURT and BRODERS reported that, of the patients with cancer treated by surgical methods at the Mayo Clinic in 1929, 3.3% had multiple primary lesions. Studying patients with malignant lesions operated on at the Mayo Clinic in 1937, STALKER and associates found that 4.5% had multiple tumors. This increasing frequency seems, from an overall study of the literature, to have continued to the present. It probably reflects the generally improved survival rate after treatment of malignant disease, in that an increased period of survival has permitted more patients to live long enough for a second primary lesion to develop, and it probably also reflects more thorough pathologic studies in both surgical and autopsy cases.

From the standpoint of numbers alone, patients with multiple primary malignant neoplasms present a significant medical problem. Of still greater import, however, is the possible contribution to the basic knowledge of malignant disease that may be afforded by a study of patients in whom two or more independent neoplasms have developed. It may be hoped that factors of genetic predisposition, etiology, and pathogenesis that are obscure in the patient with single lesions may be brought out in bolder relief in the patient with multiple cancers.

In this regard, the question of cancer immunity and predisposition has received the most attention in the literature and has engendered the least unanimity of opinion, as the following quotations witness:

A cured tumor leaves protection of the body against the development of other malignant neoplasms (PELLER).

Cases of multiple malignant growths occur more frequently than the expected incidence based on chance alone. This greater frequency, calculated as elevenfold, may be attributed to susceptibility or predisposition to cancer in some persons or groups of persons (WARREN and EHRENREICH).

... there is no demonstrable influence either of a constitutional predisposition to the development of cancer in different organs or of any immunity resulting from a first cancer (T. A. WATSON).

This remarkable contrast is but a sampling of the confusing labyrinth of statistics, controls, and conclusions through which the reader must search in an attempt to evaluate the relative incidence of multiple primary malignant neoplasms. A poignant and apropos appraisal of the statistical methodology employed in some of these studies was made by EPSTEIN, who demonstrated that by comparing his data to different control groups he could prove the incidence of a second primary cancer to be greater than, less than, or the same as that expected by chance alone. The present inadequacies in our knowledge of malignant disease and the lack of wholly reliable figures on the incidence of cancer in the general population or any segment thereof may invalidate even the most carefully chosen control group.

On the whole, the literature concerning this subject leaves the impression that the incidence of a second cancer of a different organ or tissue in patients whose first lesion has been treated successfully is probably equal to, and perhaps exceeds, that in the general population. However, convincing statistical evidence is still lacking, and because the establishment of an adequate control group for our study is not possible, no attempt at this type of analysis will be made in the present study.

1. Criteria for Diagnosis

Since the patterns of growth, local spread, and metastasis of malignant neoplasms are often bizarre and unpredictable, the criteria which distinguish a second primary lesion from a recurrence or a metastatic growth cannot be absolute. It then becomes necessary to select cases by criteria which are neither so lax that the results of a study are highly questionable nor so rigid that the practical clinical value of the study is lost.

The following criteria have been erroneously attributed to BILLROTH and perpetuated through the literature:

1. Each tumor must have a different histologic appearance.
2. The tumors must arise in different locations.
3. Each tumor must produce its own metastasis.

A careful translation of BILLROTH's writings on this subject, however, revealed that he neither stated nor implied such unrealistically rigid criteria. Indeed, one of the patients whose case he reported had two epitheliomas of the oral cavity, and in describing another of his patients he specifically stated that one of the lesions, an epithelioma of the face, showed no evidence of metastasis.

The majority of recent workers in this field have agreed that the criteria established by WARREN and GATES in 1932 are practical and realistic, and these are the criteria applied in the selection of cases for this study. These are as follows:

1. Each of the tumors must present a definite picture of malignancy.

2. Each must be distinct.

3. The probability that one was a metastatic lesion from the other must be excluded.

2. Classification

When the many specific types of malignant neoplasms to which man may fall prey are considered, the number of different combinations of multiple primary cancers seems almost countless, and a meaningful classification of these cases seems impossible. However, a review of the larger series reported in the literature discloses that in more than half of the reported cases the multiple cancers are confined to the same organ or to bilaterally paired organs. When SLAUGHTER reviewed the literature in 1944, he found multiple cancers of the same or paired organs in 1,018 (54 %) of the 1,868 cases he collected. In 57 % of the 1,010 cases in the single series of MACDONALD, and in 54 % of the 1,171 cases in the single series of WATSON, the same or paired organs were affected. Although the relative incidence of multiple neoplasms of different organs or tissues is a disputed point, almost all authors have agreed that multiple cancers of the same organ or paired organs occur far more frequently than would be expected by chance alone. This relationship is apparent to all in respect to epitheliomas of the skin, for as many as 16 % of the patients have been reported as presenting with multiple lesions (PHILLIPS). It also has been demonstrated adequately for carcinomas of the colon, breast, oral cavity, and urinary tract. These observations as well as significant histologic studies by WILLIS, SLAUGHTER (2), COLLINS and GALL, McGRATH and associates, QUALHEIM and GALL, WILLIAMS, and BLACK and ACKERMAN have led to the concept of multicentricity of origin of malignant neoplasms. This will be discussed more thoroughly in subsequent sections of this monograph.

In 1933 LUND suggested that entirely different etiologic and pathogenetic mechanisms were involved in multiple cancers of the same organ and multiple cancers of different organs or tissues. He classified his series of cases accordingly, separating those with lesions of multicentric origin from those with lesions of different tissues of origin. Later studies have tended to confirm the meaningfulness of this classification. The classification used in this study is largely an expansion of that initially proposed by Lund:

    I. Multiple primary malignant neoplasms of multicentric origin.

        A) Multicentric lesions of the same tissue and organ.

        B) Multicentric lesions of a common, contiguous tissue shared by different organs.

        C) Multicentric lesions of bilaterally paired organs.

II. Multiple primary malignant neoplasms of different tissues or organs.

III. Multiple primary malignant neoplasms of multicentric origin plus a lesion (s) of a different tissue or organ.

3. Selection of Cases for Our Study

Material for the present study is derived from the clinical and pathologic observations on all patients with histologically proved malignant neoplasms seen at the Mayo Clinic and its affiliated hospitals during the 10-year period from January 1, 1944, to December 31, 1953. Cases were included only if a pathologic examination of each lesion had been made at this clinic; patients who gave a history of a malignant neoplasm treated elsewhere were included only if a tissue specimen had been submitted to this clinic for pathologic examination. Also cases were included only if a tissue diagnosis had been made; cases in which the diagnosis was made from the cytologic smear alone were discarded.

All cases thus obtained in which the diagnosis of multiple primary malignant neoplasms had been made initially were studied further. The full clinical, surgical, and pathologic records of each patient were examined. All cases were discarded in which the malignancy of one or both lesions was considered equivocal, as in the low-grade carcinoma in situ in an adenomatous polyp or the mixed tumor of the salivary glands. Also, all cases in which each lesion was not discrete were discarded, for example cases of colliding tumors and carcinosarcomas. In all cases in which doubt existed as to whether one lesion was metastatic from the other, the pathologic material was reexamined. If after this reexamination a reasonable doubt still existed, the case was discarded.

Special attention was given to multicentric lesions. Simultaneous multicentric lesions were accepted only if they were distinctly separated by normal tissue or, in cases of interval lesions, only if the most recent lesion was distinctly separated from the site of excision of the initial lesion, regardless of the time intervening between the diagnosis of the two neoplasms. Multiple epitheliomas confined to the skin alone were not included in this study, because the frequent multicentricity of these lesions is obvious and well documented and their inclusion would serve no purpose except to increase needlessly the total number of cases studied.

Every effort was made to ensure that the cases included represented true multiple primary malignant neoplasms beyond any reasonable doubt. It became obvious as our work progressed that such careful attention to case selection was essential to the validity of a study of this kind. A large number of cases originally classified as multiple primary cancers were discarded on review, because they quite clearly represented examples of regional spread or distant metastasis from a solitary primary lesion. To conduct a study of multiple primary cancers by using only tumor registry data without a careful pathologic review may open the door to gross distortion of results.

4. Observations

During the 10-year period from January 1, 1944, to December 31, 1953, a total of 1,909 patients had been given a diagnosis of multiple primary malignant neoplasms at the Mayo Clinic, and this diagnosis met the criteria previously mentioned. This group was composed of 1,172 males and 737 females. In 1,663 patients, all lesions were diagnosed at operation; in 95, all lesions were diagnosed at autopsy; and in 151, lesions were diagnosed both at operation and at autopsy. Eight hundred and forty-one patients (596 males, 245 females) had lesions which were diagnosed simultaneously; 983 patients (522 males and 461 females) had lesions diagnosed at an interval; and 85 patients (54 males and 31 females) had both simultaneous and interval lesions[1].

Of those patients with interval lesions, 989 had two consecutive neoplasms; 74 had three consecutive neoplasms; 4 had four consecutive neoplasms; and 1 patient had five consecutive neoplasms. The average interval between the first and second cancers was 6.9 years (6.4 years for male patients, 7.7 years for female patients) with a range of 6 months to 36 years. The multiple lesions were diagnosed simultaneously in almost half of the patients in this series; and, as can be seen in Fig. 1,

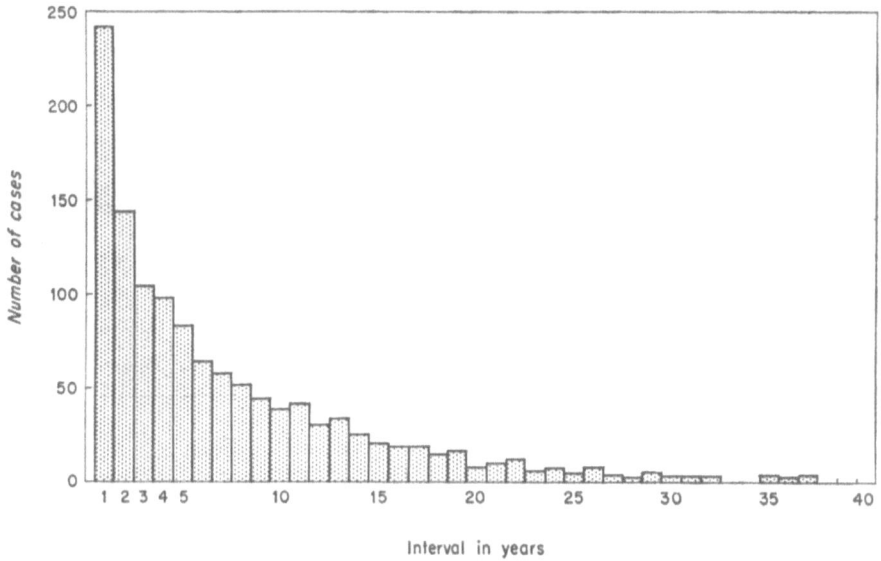

Fig. 1 Interval between diagnosis of lesions of patients with nonsynchronous multiple primary malignant neoplasms. (From MOERTEL, C. G., M. B. DOCKERTY, and A. H. BAGGENSTOSS: Multiple primary malignant neoplasms. I. Introduction and presentation of data. Cancer [Philad.] 14, 221 [1961]. By permission of the publisher, J. B. Lippincott Company)

the number of patients with interval cancers decreased in a logarithmic fashion with the passage of time after the diagnosis of the initial lesion. Undoubtedly many factors contribute to this temporal relationship, but from a practical point of view it should be mentioned that the time when second primary cancers have been observed most frequently is the time when the clinician is most likely to be misled by the possibility of metastasis or recurrence.

The average age and range of ages of the patients in this series are presented in Table 1. The youngest patient in this series, and apparently the youngest to be

---

[1] All lesions diagnosed within the same 6-month period were arbitrarily classified as "simultaneous lesions"; all lesions diagnosed at intervals of longer than 6 months were classified as "interval lesions."

reported in the literature, is a 14-month-old child who was found at autopsy to have an astrocytoma of the spinal cord as well as an extradural fibromyxosarcoma of the thoracic portion of the spinal column. DODGE and associates have reported

Table 1. *Age of Patients at the Time of Diagnosis of Multiple Primary Malignant Neoplasms*

	Age of male patients, yr		Age of female patients, yr	
	Average	Range	Average	Range
Simultaneous lesions	62.0	1 to 93	58.0	17 to 85
Interval lesions:				
Initial lesion	57.0	10 to 89	51.3	20 to 61
Second lesion	63.4	14 to 91	59.2	25 to 88
Third lesion	66.8	36 to 85	63.3	48 to 85

this case. The oldest patient was a 93-year-old man who was found at autopsy to have a squamous cell carcinoma of the mouth, an adenocarcinoma of the stomach, and an adenocarcinoma of the prostate.

5. Rate of Occurrence

During the 10-year period of this study, a total of 37,580 patients had malignant neoplasms pathologically verified at this clinic either at the time of operation or at autopsy. Thus, the 1,909 patients found to have multiple primary malignant neoplasms represent an overall rate of occurrence of 5.1 %. This rate of occurrence is broken down in more detail in Table 2.

Table 2. *Rate of Occurrence of Multiple Primary Malignant Neoplasms* [1]

	Patients with proved cancer	Multiple primary cancers In all tissues		In different tissues	
		Patients	Rate of occurrence, %	Patients	Rate of occurrence, %
Surgical cases					
Male	21,368	998	4.7	539	2.5
Female	15,179	676	4.5	302	2.0
Total	36,547	1,674	4.6	841	2.3
Autopsy cases [2]					
Male	1,907	218	11.4	184	9.7
Female	995	91	9.1	52	5.2
Total	2,902	309	10.6	236	8.1
All cases:					
Surgical and autopsy					
Male	22,054	1,172	5.3	701	3.2
Female	15,526	737	4.8	348	2.2
Total	37,580	1,909	5.1	1,049	2.8

[1] Exclusive of patients with multiple epitheliomas confined to the skin alone.
[2] Includes all patients coming to autopsy with multiple primary malignant neoplasms proved either before or at autopsy.

Although statistics for the rate of occurrence of multiple primary malignant tumors are commonly expressed in this fashion in the literature, such figures are of limited value since they represent a mixture of two decidedly different occurrence rates — that for multiple lesions of different organs or tissues and that for lesions of multicentric origin. To have significance, the occurrence rates should be expressed individually. In Table 2 the occurrence rates for multiple primary cancers of different tissues or organs are presented. The occurrence rates of multicentric neoplasms will be given later when the specific organs involved are discussed.

It is readily apparent that the incidence of multiple malignant neoplasms found at autopsy far exceeds that found clinically. This increase is in large part the result of lesions discovered as "incidental" autopsy findings — that is, lesions which produced no signs or symptoms during life and in no way contributed to death. Of the 309 patients with multiple primary cancers who came to autopsy, 121 patients (39%) had one or more lesions which could be considered as incidental findings. It also should be brought out that if it may be assumed that the incidence of incidental malignant neoplasms is the same in patients dying of either malignant or nonmalignant disease, then the incidence of multiple malignant neoplasms will be higher in an institution such as the Mayo Clinic, where a relatively large number of patients with malignant disease as a cause or a contributing cause of death come to autopsy.

It must be emphasized that the rate of occurrence of multiple primary cancers given herein is undoubtedly significantly less than the actual incidence. Many patients were seen who gave a history of a malignant neoplasm treated elsewhere before their visit to this clinic, but material was not available for pathologic confirmation at this clinic, hence these patients were not included in the present study. Also it seems likely that many patients treated successfully at this clinic for an initial cancer may have had subsequent malignant neoplasms for which they were treated elsewhere or which were present and untreated at the time of their later death.

Even if all the patients with multiple primary malignant neoplasms could be tabulated, the incidence as calculated in this paper would still be deceptively low. A high percentage of patients with proved cancer succumb to the initial lesion and, therefore, do not live long enough for a second cancer to develop even if they might have been so destined. If future advances in cancer therapy bring about a progressively larger percentage of long-term survivals, the proportion of cancer patients who will fall victim to a second primary lesion doubtless will increase.

When a patient has been found to have multiple primary cancers of different tissues of origin, does this establish him as a "cancer prone" individual, and is he

Table 3. *Rate of Occurrence of Additional Cancers in Patients With Single Cancers and in Patients With Multiple Cancers of Different Tissues of Origin*

Number of cancers	Patients	Patients with additional cancers	Rate of occurrence
1	37,580	1,049	2.8%
2	1,049	52	5.0%
3	52	3	5.8%

more likely to experience additional malignant neoplasms than the patient who has only had a single lesion? The data in Table 3 would seem to answer this question in the affirmative. The incidence of second cancers in the patient who has had a single malignant neoplasm is only 2.8 %, whereas the incidence of a third primary cancer in patients known to have had two is 5.0 %, and the incidence of a fourth primary lesion in patients with three rises to 5.8 % — this in spite of the fact that the patient's chance of surviving to acquire another lesion is decreased progressively by each cancer.

Patients in whom multiple primary cancers of different tissues of origin have developed should be considered as having a high susceptibility to neoplasia. They should be frequently and carefully reexamined with all practical screening tests for malignant disease.

6. Report of Cases

In Tables 4, 5, and 6 the specific combinations of malignant neoplasms found in the patients in this series are classified and arranged in order of frequency of occurrence within each classification. The term "epithelioma" is used collectively for both squamous cell and basal cell carcinomas of the skin and lips, and also collectively for both squamous cell and transitional cell carcinomas of the urinary tract.

Table 4. *Multiple Primary Malignant Neoplasms: I. Multicentric Origin*

Site and type of malignant neoplasms	Cases	
Confined to same tissue	(455 cases)	
Colon and rectum, ACA[1]		239
2 lesions	204	
3 lesions	20	
4 lesions	12	
5 lesions	3	
Lips, epitheliomas		63
2 lesions	56	
3 lesions	7	
Stomach, ACA		38
2 lesions	28	
3 lesions	10	
Bladder, epitheliomas		32
2 lesions	23	
3 lesions	7	
4 lesions	2	
Mouth, SCE[1]		1
2 lesions	17	6
3 lesions	2	
Larynx, SCE — 2 lesions		15

[1] ACA = adenocarcinoma; SCE = squamous cell epithelioma.

Site and type of malignant neoplasms	Cases	
Tongue, SCE		11
2 lesions	10	
3 lesions	1	
Brain, astrocytomas		10
2 lesions	7	
3 lesions	3	
Ileum, carcinoids		8
2 lesions	1	
3 lesions	2	
Many lesions	5	
Kidney pelvis, unilateral		4
2 lesions	1	
Multiple lesions	3	
Kidney, hypernephroma, unilateral — 2 lesions		3
Ureter, epitheliomas		3
2 lesions	2	
4 lesions	1	
Vulva, SCE — 2 lesions		3
Gallbladder, ACA — 2 lesions		2
Uterus, endometrium, ACA — 2 lesions		2
Brain ependymomas — 3 lesions		1
Esophagus, SCE — 3 lesions		1
Stomach, leiomyosarcomas — 2 lesions		1
Involving a common, contiguous tissue shared by different organs	(287 cases)	
Lips and skin, epitheliomas		148
Lip — 1 lesion + skin — 1 lesion	77	
Lip — 1 lesion + skin — multiple lesions	56	
Lips — 2 lesions + skin — 1 lesion	6	
Lips — 2 lesions + skin — multiple lesions	9	
Mouth, tongue, pharynx, larynx and esophagus, SCE, and lips, epitheliomas		89
Larynx — 1 lesion + lip — 1 lesion	4	
Larynx — 1 lesion + lips — 2 lesions	1	
Larynx — 1 lesion + mouth — 1 lesion	8	
Larynx — 2 lesions + mouth — 1 lesion	1	
Larynx — 1 lesion + pharynx — 1 lesion	1	
Larynx — 1 lesion + tongue — 1 lesion	1	
Larynx — 2 lesions + esophagus — 1 lesion	1	
Lip — 1 lesion + mouth — 1 lesion	20	
Lip — 1 lesion + mouth — 2 lesions	3	
Lip — 1 lesion + mouth — 3 lesions	1	

Table 4 (continued)

Site and type of malignant neoplasms	Cases	
Lips — 2 lesions + mouth — 1 lesion	1	
Lips — 3 lesions + mouth — 1 lesion	1	
Lip — 1 lesion + pharynx — 1 lesion	3	
Lip — 1 lesion + tongue — 1 lesion	2	
Mouth — 1 lesion + pharynx — 1 lesion	4	
Mouth — 1 lesion + tongue — 1 lesion	13	
Mouth — 1 lesion + tongue — 2 lesions	4	
Mouth — 2 lesions + tongue — 1 lesion	6	
Mouth — 2 lesions + tongue — 2 lesions	1	
Mouth — 1 lesion + esophagus — 1 lesion	2	
Pharynx — 1 lesion + esophagus — 1 lesion	2	
Pharynx — 1 lesion + tongue — 1 lesion	2	
Tongue — 1 lesion + esophagus — 1 lesion	2	
Larynx — 1 lesion + mouth — 1 lesion + tongue — 1 lesion	1	
Larynx — 1 lesion + mouth — 1 lesion + esophagus — 1 lesion	1	
Lips — 2 lesions + mouth — 1 lesion + tongue — 2 lesions	1	
Lips — 2 lesions + mouth — 2 lesions + tongue — 1 lesion	1	
Mouth — 1 lesion + pharynx — 1 lesion + tongue — 1 lesion	1	
Bladder, kidney pelvis, ureter and urethra, epitheliomas		39
Bladder — 1 lesion + kidney pelvis — 1 lesion	15	
Bladder — 1 lesion + kidney pelvis — 2 lesions	1	
Bladder — 2 lesions + kidney pelvis — 1 lesion	2	
Bladder — 1 lesion + ureter — 1 lesion	4	
Bladder — 1 lesion + urethra — 1 lesion	4	
Bladder — 2 lesions + urethra — 1 lesion	1	
Kidney pelvis — multiple lesions + ureter — 1 lesion	2	
Kidney pelvis — 1 lesion + ureter — 1 lesion	3	
Kidney pelvis — 1 lesion + ureter — 3 lesions	1	
Bladder — 1 lesion + kidney pelvis — 1 lesion + ureter — 1 lesion	4	
Bladder — 1 lesion + kidney pelvis — 1 lesion + ureter — 3 lesions	1	
Bladder — 3 lesions + kidney pelvis — 1 lesion + urethra — 1 lesion	1	
Cervix, vagina, vulva and anus, SCE		10
Cervix — 1 lesion + vulva — 1 lesion	4	
Cervix — 1 lesion + vulva — 2 lesions	1	
Cervix — 1 lesion + vulva — 3 lesions	1	
Vagina — 1 lesion + vulva — 2 lesions	2	
Vulva — 1 lesion + anus — 1 lesion	1	
Cervix — 1 lesion + vagina — 1 lesion + vulva — 1 lesion	1	
Brain and spinal cord, astrocytomas		1
Brain — multiple lesions + spinal cord — 1 lesion	1	
In bilaterally paired organs	(118 cases)	
Breasts, adenocarcinomas, bilateral		113
Testes, seminomas, bilateral		3
Kidneys, hypernephromas, bilateral		1
Ovaries, carcinomas, bilateral		1

Table 5. *Multiple Primary Malignant Neoplasms: II. Multiple Tissues of Origin*

Site and type of malignant neoplasms		Cases
Two lesions		(921 cases)
Colon, ACA[1]	Skin, epithelioma	43
Bladder, epithelioma	Prostate, ACA	40
Breast, ACA	Skin, epithelioma	30
Breast, ACA	Uterine endometrium, ACA	30
Colon, ACA	Prostate, ACA	30
Colon, ACA	Breast, ACA	28
Larynx, SCE[1]	Skin, epithelioma	22
Colon, ACA	Stomach, ACA	17
Prostate, ACA	Skin, epithelioma	17
Bladder, epithelioma	Colon, ACA	16
Colon, ACA	Lip, epithelioma	16
Colon, ACA	Uterine endometrium, ACA	16
Breast, ACA	Cervix, SCE	14
Prostate, ACA	Stomach, ACA	14
Stomach, ACA	Skin, epithelioma	14
Bladder, epithelioma	Skin, epithelioma	13
Breast, ACA	Ovary, ACA	12
Cervix, SCE	Skin, epithelioma	11
Kidney, hypernephroma	Prostate, ACA	11
Mouth, SCE	Skin, epithelioma	9
Breast, ACA	Thyroid, ACA	7
Lung, SCE	Prostate, ACA	7
Ovary, ACA	Uterine endometrium, ACA	7
Cervix, SCE	Colon, ACA	6
Colon, ACA	Kidney, hypernephroma	6
Colon, ACA	Lung, SCE	6
Colon, ACA	Skin, multiple epitheliomas	6
Lip, epithelioma	Prostate, ACA	6
Lip, epithelioma	Stomach, ACA	6
Bladder, epithelioma	Breast, ACA	5
Colon, ACA	Larynx, SCE	5
Colon, ACA	Lymphosarcoma	5
Lung, SCE	Skin, epithelioma	5
Lymphosarcoma	Skin, epithelioma	5
Prostate, ACA	Skin, multiple epitheliomas	5
Tongue, SCE	Skin, epithelioma	5
Bladder, epithelioma	Lip, epithelioma	4
Breast, ACA	Leukemia, chronic lymphatic	4
Breast, ACA	Stomach, ACA	4
Cervix, SCE	Ovary, ACA	4
Cervix, SCE	Uterine endometrium, ACA	4
Colon, ACA	Ileum, carcinoid	4
Colon, ACA	Ovary, ACA	4
Larynx, SCE	Prostate, ACA	4
Leukemia, chronic lymphatic	Skin, epithelioma	4
Ovary, ACA	Skin, epithelioma	4
Pancreas, ACA	Skin, epithelioma	4
Thyroid, ACA	Uterine endometrium, ACA	4
Bladder, epithelioma	Kidney, hypernephroma	3
Bladder, epithelioma	Lung, ACA	3
Bladder, epithelioma	Lung, SCE	3

[1] ACA = adenocarcinoma; SCE = squamous cell epithelioma.

Table 5 (continued)

Site and type of malignant neoplasms		Cases
Bladder, epithelioma	Lymphosarcoma	3
Bladder, epithelioma	Uterine endometrium, ACA	3
Brain, astrocytoma	Prostate, ACA	3
Breast, ACA	Multiple myeloma	3
Breast, ACA	Neurofibrosarcoma	3
Breast, ACA	Lymphosarcoma	3
Cervix, SCE	Pancreas, ACA	3
Colon, ACA	Hodgkin's disease	3
Colon, ACA	Lung, ACA	3
Colon, ACA	Pancreas, ACA	3
Colon, ACA	Hepatic or common bile duct, ACA	3
Kidney, hypernephroma	Pancreas, ACA	3
Leukemia, chronic lymphatic	Stomach, ACA	3
Leukemia, chronic lymphatic	Skin, multiple epitheliomas	3
Leukemia, chronic lymphatic	Prostate, ACA	3
Lip, epithelioma	Lymphosarcoma	3
Lip, epithelioma	Thyroid, ACA	3
Lymphosarcoma	Skin, multiple epitheliomas	3
Multiple myeloma	Prostate, ACA	3
Pancreas, ACA	Stomach, ACA	3
Pharynx, SCE	Prostate, ACA	3
Reticulum cell sarcoma	Skin, epithelioma	3
Uterus, ACA	Skin, epithelioma	3
Appendix, ACA	Colon, ACA	2
Appendix, ACA	Uterine endometrium, ACA	2
Bladder, epithelioma	Cervix, SCE	2
Bladder, epithelioma	Fibromyxosarcoma	2
Bladder, epithelioma	Leukemia, chronic lymphatic	2
Bladder, epithelioma	Mouth, SCE	2
Bladder, epithelioma	Stomach, ACA	2
Bladder, epithelioma	Thyroid, ACA	2
Breast, ACA	Esophagus, SCE	2
Breast, ACA	Leukemia, chronic myelogenous	2
Breast, ACA	Lip, epithelioma	2
Breast, ACA	Lung, ACA	2
Breast, ACA	Skin, multiple epitheliomas	2
Breast, ACA	Vulva, SCE	2
Cervix, ACA	Ovary, ACA	2
Cervix, SCE	Larynx, SCE	2
Colon, ACA	Esophagus, SCE	2
Colon, ACA	Fibrosarcoma	2
Colon, ACA	Gallbladder, ACA	2
Colon, ACA	Kidney pelvis, epithelioma	2
Colon, ACA	Leukemia, acute lymphatic	2
Colon, ACA	Leukemia, acute myelogenous	2
Colon, ACA	Mouth, SCE	2
Colon, ACA	Thyroid, ACA	2
Colon, ACA	Tongue, SCE	2
Colon, ACA	Vulva, SCE	2
Fibrosarcoma	Lip, epithelioma	2
Gallbladder, ACA	Prostate, ACA	2
Kidney, hypernephroma	Leukemia, chronic lymphatic	2
Kidney, hypernephroma	Lung, small cell carcinoma	2
Kidney, hypernephroma	Stomach, ACA	2

Table 5 (continued)

Site and type of malignant neoplasms		Cases
Kidney pelvis, epithelioma	Prostate, ACA	2
Larynx, SCE	Lung, SCE	2
Larynx, SCE	Skin, multiple epitheliomas	2
Larynx, SCE	Thyroid, ACA	2
Leukemia, chronic myelogenous	Skin, epithelioma	2
Lip, SCE	Lung, SCE	2
Lip, SCE	Malignant melanoma	2
Lung, ACA	Prostate, ACA	2
Lung, ACA	Skin, epithelioma	2
Lung, mixed ACA and SCE	Tongue, SCE	2
Lung, SCE	Mouth, SCE	2
Lung, SCE	Skin, multiple epitheliomas	2
Lymphosarcoma	Penis, SCE	2
Lymphosarcoma	Prostate, ACA	2
Mouth, SCE	Prostate, ACA	2
Mouth, SCE	Skin, multiple epitheliomas	2
Ovary, ACA	Skin, multiple epitheliomas	2
Pancreas, ACA	Prostate, ACA	2
Pancreas, ACA	Thyroid, ACA	2
Pancreas, ACA	Uterine endometrium, ACA	2
Stomach, ACA	Skin, multiple epitheliomas	2
Stomach, ACA	Thyroid, ACA	2
Uterus, ACA	Uterus, leiomyosarcoma	2
Adrenal, ACA	Malignant melanoma	1
Ampulla of Vater, ACA	Prostate, ACA	1
Angiosarcoma	Breast, ACA	1
Anus, basal cell carcinoma	Prostate, ACA	1
Anus, SCE	Uterine endometrium, ACA	1
Appendix, ACA	Ovary, ACA	1
Appendix, ACA	Skin, epithelioma	1
Appendix, carcinoid	Ovary, ACA	1
Appendix, carcinoid	Uterine endometrium, ACA	1
Bladder, epithelioma	Cervix, ACA	1
Bladder, epithelioma	Fibrosarcoma	1
Bladder, epithelioma	Jejunum, ACA	1
Bladder, epithelioma	Larynx, SCE	1
Bladder, epithelioma	Leiomyosarcoma	1
Bladder, epithelioma	Leukemia, chronic myelogenous	1
Bladder, epithelioma	Malignant melanoma	1
Bladder, epithelioma	Multiple myeloma	1
Bladder, epithelioma	Ovary, ACA	1
Bladder, epithelioma	Pancreas, ACA	1
Bladder, epithelioma	Pancreas, islet cell carcinoma	1
Bladder, epithelioma	Penis, SCE	1
Bladder, epithelioma	Pharynx, SCE	1
Bladder, epithelioma	Skin, multiple epitheliomas	1
Bladder, epithelioma	Tongue, SCE	1
Bone, Ewing's tumor	Skin, epithelioma	1
Bone, osteogenic sarcoma	Hemangio-endothelioma	1
Bone, osteogenic sarcoma	Skin, multiple epitheliomas	1
Bone, unclassifiable	Leukemia, chronic lymphatic	1
Brain, astrocytoma	Brain, hemangio-endothelioma	1
Brain, astrocytoma	Breast, ACA	1
Brain, astrocytoma	Colon, ACA	1

Table 5 (continued)

Site and type of malignant neoplasms		Cases
Brain, astrocytoma	Jejunum, ACA	1
Brain, astrocytoma	Pancreas, ACA	1
Brain, astrocytoma	Reticulum cell sarcoma	1
Brain, astrocytoma	Stomach, ACA	1
Brain, astrocytoma	Brain, mixed oligodendroglioma and ependymoma	1
Breast, ACA	Cervix, ACA	1
Breast, ACA	Eyelid, ACA	1
Breast, ACA	Giant cell sarcoma	1
Breast, ACA	Hodgkin's disease	1
Breast, ACA	Ileum, carcinoid	1
Breast, ACA	Larynx, SCE	1
Breast, ACA	Liver, ACA	1
Breast, ACA	Mastoid, malignant chemodectoma	1
Breast, ACA	Malignant melanoma	1
Breast, ACA	Mouth, ACA	1
Breast, ACA	Pancreas, ACA	1
Breast, ACA	Paranasal sinus, sarcoma	1
Breast, ACA	Parotid, ACA	1
Breast, ACA	Pharynx, SCE	1
Breast, ACA	Rectum, SCE	1
Breast, ACA	Urethra, epithelioma	1
Breast, ACA	Uterus, leiomyosarcoma	1
Cauda equina, malignant neurilemmoma	Leukemia, acute myelogenous	1
Cervix, ACA	Colon, ACA	1
Cervix, ACA	Lymphosarcoma	1
Cervix, ACA	Uterine endometrium, ACA	1
Cervix, SCE	Kidney pelvis, epithelioma	1
Cervix, SCE	Liposarcoma	1
Cervix, SCE	Lymphosarcoma	1
Cervix, SCE	Pharynx, SCE	1
Cervix, SCE	Reticulum cell sarcoma	1
Cervix, SCE	Stomach, ACA	1
Cervix, SCE	Stomach, leiomyosarcoma	1
Cervix, SCE	Thyroid, ACA	1
Cervix, SCE	Urethra, epithelioma	1
Colon, ACA	Esophagus, ACA	1
Colon, ACA	Hemangio-endothelioma	1
Colon, ACA	Jejunum, ACA	1
Colon, ACA	Leukemia, acute lymphatic	1
Colon, ACA	Liposarcoma	1
Colon, ACA	Multiple myeloma	1
Colon, ACA	Pancreas, SCE	1
Colon, ACA	Parotid, ACA	1
Colon, ACA	Sarcoma, unclassified	1
Colon, ACA	Stomach, leiomyosarcoma	1
Colon, ACA	Unclassified anaplastic neoplasm	1
Colon, ACA	Urethra, ACA	1
Colon, ACA	Urethra, epithelioma	1
Common bile duct, ACA	Prostate, ACA	1
Epididymis, carcinoma sarcomatoides	Stomach, ACA	1
Esophagus, ACA	Leukemia, chronic lymphatic	1
Esophagus, ACA	Skin, epithelioma	1

Table 5 (continued)

Site and type of malignant neoplasms		Cases
Esophagus, SCE	Fibrosarcoma	1
Esophagus, SCE	Kidney pelvis, epithelioma	1
Esophagus, SCE	Lymphosarcoma	1
Esophagus, SCE	Skin, epithelioma	1
Fibromyxosarcoma	Ovary, ACA	1
Fibromyxosarcoma	Spinal cord, astrocytoma	1
Fibrosarcoma	Lung, SCE	1
Fibrosarcoma	Mouth, SCE	1
Fibrosarcoma	Nasal fossa, ACA	1
Fibrosarcoma	Skin, epithelioma	1
Hemangio-endothelioma	Paranasal sinus, ACA	1
Hemangio-endothelioma	Paranasal sinus, SCE	1
Hemangio-endothelioma	Skin, epithelioma	1
Hodgkin's disease	Lip, epithelioma	1
Hodgkin's disease	Lung, ACA	1
Hodgkin's disease	Pharynx, SCE	1
Hodgkin's disease	Prostate, ACA	1
Hodgkin's disease	Ovary, ACA	1
Hodgkin's disease	Skin, epithelioma	1
Hodgkin's disease	Stomach, ACA	1
Hodgkin's disease	Thyroid, ACA	1
Hodgkin's disease	Uterine endometrium, ACA	1
Ileum, carcinoid	Prostate, ACA	1
Ileum, carcinoid	Stomach, ACA	1
Ileum, carcinoid	Tongue, SCE	1
Jejunum, carcinoid	Stomach, ACA	1
Kaposi's sarcoma	Mouth, SCE	1
Kaposi's sarcoma	Lymphosarcoma	1
Kaposi's sarcoma	Skin, epithelioma	1
Kidney, hypernephroma	Leiomyosarcoma	1
Kidney, hypernephroma	Lip, epithelioma	1
Kidney, hypernephroma	Liver, ACA	1
Kidney, hypernephroma	Ovary, ACA	1
Kidney, hypernephroma	Pharynx, SCE	1
Kidney, hypernephroma	Stomach, leiomyosarcoma	1
Kidney, hypernephroma	Ureter, epithelioma	1
Kidney, hypernephroma	Uterine endometrium, ACA	1
Kidney pelvis, epithelioma	Ovary, ACA	1
Kidney pelvis, epithelioma	Stomach, ACA	1
Larynx, SCE	Leukemia, chronic lymphatic	1
Larynx, SCE	Malignant melanoma	1
Larynx, SCE	Paranasal sinus, SCE	1
Larynx, SCE	Vulva, SCE	1
Leukemia, acute monocytic	Prostate, SCE	1
Leukemia, acute myelogenous	Stomach, ACA	1
Leukemia, acute myelogenous	Testis, seminoma	1
Leukemia, acute stem cell	Skin, multiple epitheliomas	1
Leukemia, chronic lymphatic	Lip, epithelioma	1
Leukemia, chronic lymphatic	Lung, ACA	1
Leukemia, chronic lymphatic	Lung, SCE	1
Leukemia, chronic lymphatic	Uterus, SCE	1
Leukemia, chronic myelogenous	Lip, epithelioma	1
Leukemia, chronic myelogenous	Lung, ACA	1
Leukemia, chronic myelogenous	Prostate, ACA	1

Table 5 (continued)

Site and type of malignant neoplasms		Cases
Leukemia, chronic myelogenous	Pharynx, SCE	1
Lip, ACA	Lymphosarcoma	1
Lip, epithelioma	Lung, ACA	1
Lip, epithelioma	Mouth, ACA	1
Lip, epithelioma	Urethra, epithelioma	1
Lung, ACA	Malignant melanoma	1
Lung, ACA	Skin, multiple epitheliomas	1
Lung, SCE	Ovary, ACA	1
Lung, SCE	Pancreas, ACA	1
Lung, SCE	Stomach, ACA	1
Lung, SCE	Testis, seminoma	1
Lung, SCE	Thyroid, ACA	1
Lymphosarcoma	Mouth, SCE	1
Lymphosarcoma	Ovary, ACA	1
Lymphosarcoma	Stomach, ACA	1
Lymphosarcoma	Testis, teratocarcinoma	1
Lymphosarcoma	Thyroid, ACA	1
Lymphosarcoma	Uterus, ACA	1
Malignant melanoma	Prostate, ACA	1
Malignant melanoma	Skin, multiple epitheliomas	1
Mouth, SCE	Pancreas, ACA	1
Mouth, SCE	Skin, epithelioma	1
Mouth, SCE	Uterine endometrium, ACA	1
Nasal fossa, SCE	Skin, epithelioma	1
Ovary, ACA	Ovary, leiomyosarcoma	1
Ovary, ACA	Thyroid, ACA	1
Ovary, theca cell sarcoma	Uterus, mixed ACA and fibromyxosarcoma	1
Paranasal sinus, SCE	Skin, epithelioma	1
Parotid, ACA	Skin, epithelioma	1
Parotid, SCE	Pharynx, SCE	1
Parotid, SCE	Thyroid, ACA	1
Penis, SCE	Prostate, ACA	1
Penis, SCE	Skin, epithelioma	1
Pharynx, SCE	Skin, multiple epitheliomas	1
Prostate, ACA	Reticulum cell sarcoma	1
Prostate, ACA	Rhabdomyosarcoma	1
Prostate, ACA	Trachea, ACA	1
Rectum, carcinoid	Testis, carcinoma	1
Reticulum cell sarcoma	Stomach, ACA	1
Stomach, ACA	Stomach, leiomyosarcoma	1
Stomach, ACA	Testis, seminoma	1
Stomach, ACA	Tongue, SCE	1
Stomach, ACA	Uterine endometrium, ACA	1
Submaxillary gland, SCE	Skin, epithelioma	1
Testis, seminoma	Skin, epithelioma	1
Testis, seminoma	Testis, teratocarcinoma	1
Thyroid, ACA	Skin, epithelioma	1
Thyroid, ACA	Skin, multiple epitheliomas	1
Tongue, SCE	Skin, multiple epitheliomas	1
Tongue, SCE	Uterus, leiomyosarcoma	1
Urethra, epithelioma	Uterus, fibromyxosarcoma	1
Uterus, ACA	Uterus, hemangio-endothelioma	1
Uterus, ACA	Vagina, SCE	1
Vulva, SCE	Skin, epithelioma	1

Table 5 (continued)

Site and type of malignant neoplasms			Cases
Vulva, SCE	Skin, multiple epitheliomas		1
Three lesions			(46 cases)
Bladder, epithelioma	Prostate, ACA	Skin, epithelioma	2
Colon, ACA	Leukemia, chronic myelogenous	Skin, epithelioma	2
Colon, ACA	Prostate, ACA	Skin, multiple epitheliomas	2
Bladder, epithelioma	Kidney, hypernephroma	Prostate, ACA	1
Bladder, epithelioma	Lip, epithelioma	Prostate, ACA	1
Bladder, epithelioma	Prostate, ACA	Stomach, ACA	1
Brain, astrocytoma	Prostate, ACA	Stomach, ACA	1
Brain, malignant meningioma	Malignant melanoma	Skin, multiple epitheliomas	1
Breast, ACA	Cervix, SCE	Colon, ACA	1
Breast, ACA	Colon, ACA	Uterus, ACA	1
Breast, ACA	Gallbladder, ACA	Ovary, ACA	1
Breast, ACA	Ovary, ACA	Pancreas, ACA	1
Breast, ACA	Ovary, ACA	Uterine endometrium, ACA	1
Breast, ACA	Neurofibrosarcoma	Skin, multiple epitheliomas	1
Breast, ACA	Thyroid, ACA	Skin, multiple epitheliomas	1
Breast, ACA	Uterine endometrium, ACA	Skin, epithelioma	1
Cervix, SCE	Larynx, SCE	Skin, epithelioma	1
Colon, ACA	Esophagus, ACA	Prostate, ACA	1
Colon, ACA	Fibrosarcoma	Skin, epithelioma	1
Colon, ACA	Kidney, hypernephroma	Thyroid, ACA	1
Colon, ACA	Kidney pelvis, epithelioma	Prostate, ACA	1
Colon, ACA	Lip, epithelioma	Prostate, ACA	1
Colon, ACA	Lymphosarcoma	Skin, epithelioma	1
Colon, ACA	Ovary, granulosa cell carcinoma	Uterine endometrium, ACA	1
Colon, ACA	Pancreas, ACA	Skin, epithelioma	1
Colon, ACA	Pancreas, ACA	Stomach, ACA	1
Colon, ACA	Stomach, ACA	Tongue, SCE	1
Duodenum, carcinoid	Prostate, ACA	Stomach, ACA	1
Kaposi's sarcoma	Lymphosarcoma	Prostate, ACA	1
Kidney, hypernephroma	Lip, epithelioma	Stomach, ACA	1
Kidney, hypernephroma	Mouth, SCE	Prostate, ACA	1
Kidney, hypernephroma	Prostate, ACA	Skin, epithelioma	1
Kidney, hypernephroma	Prostate, ACA	Stomach, ACA	1
Lip, ACA	Tongue, SCE	Skin, epithelioma	1
Lip, epithelioma	Lung, SCE	Prostate, ACA	1
Leukemia, chronic lymphatic	Prostate, ACA	Skin, epithelioma	1
Lung, SCE	Mouth, SCE	Skin, epithelioma	1
Lung, SCE	Multiple myeloma	Skin, epithelioma	1
Lung, SCE	Pancreas, ACA	Skin, epithelioma	1
Lung, SCE	Prostate, ACA	Thyroid, ACA	1
Lymphosarcoma	Malignant melanoma	Skin, epithelioma	1
Ovary, ACA	Pancreas, ACA	Stomach, ACA	1
Ovary, ACA	Thyroid, ACA	Uterine endometrium, ACA	1
Four lesions			(1 case)
Ovary, granulosa cell carcinoma + uterine endometrium, ACA + uterus, leiomyosarcoma + skin, epithelioma			1
Five lesions			(1 case)
Breast, ACA + colon, ACA + skin, epithelioma + ureter, SCE + uterine endometrium, ACA			1

Table 6. *Multiple Primary Malignant Neoplasms: III. Multicentric Malignant Neoplasms Plus One or More Malignant Neoplasms of Different Tissues of Origin*

Site and type of malignant neoplasms	Cases
Colon and rectum, ACA[1] + other	24
Colon and rectum, ACA — 2 lesions + skin, epithelioma	3
Colon and rectum, ACA — 2 lesions + breast, ACA	2
Colon and rectum, ACA — 2 lesions + prostate, ACA	2
Colon and rectum, ACA — 2 lesions + bladder, epithelioma	1
Colon and rectum, ACA — 2 lesions + ileum, ACA	1
Colon and rectum, ACA — 2 lesions + ileum, carcinoid	1
Colon and rectum, ACA — 2 lesions + fibrosarcoma	1
Colon and rectum, ACA — 2 lesions + hepatic duct, ACA	1
Colon and rectum, ACA — 2 lesions + larynx, SCE[1]	1
Colon and rectum, ACA — 2 lesions + leukemia, acute lymphatic	1
Colon and rectum, ACA — 2 lesions + ovary, ACA	1
Colon and rectum, ACA — 2 lesions + stomach, ACA	1
Colon and rectum, ACA — 2 lesions + uterus, ACA	1
Colon and rectum, ACA — 3 lesions + breast, ACA	1
Colon and rectum, ACA — 3 lesions + ileum, many carcinoids	1
Colon and rectum, ACA — 4 lesions + bladder, epithelioma	2
Colon and rectum, ACA — 4 lesions + jejunum, ACA	1
Colon and rectum, ACA — 4 lesions + ovary, ACA	1
Colon and rectum, ACA — 4 lesions + vulva, SCE + lymphosarcoma	1
Lips and skin, epitheliomas + other	17
Lip — 1 lesion + skin — 1 lesion + colon, ACA	4
Lip — 1 lesion + skin — 1 lesion + mouth, SCE	2
Lip — 1 lesion + skin — 1 lesion + bladder, epithelioma	1
Lip — 1 lesion + skin — 1 lesion + larynx, SCE	1
Lip — 1 lesion + skin — 1 lesion + malignant melanoma	1
Lip — 1 lesion + skin — 1 lesion + tongue, SCE	1
Lip — 1 lesion + skin — multiple lesions + colon, ACA	2
Lip — 1 lesion + skin — multiple lesions + cervix, SCE	1
Lip — 1 lesion + skin — multiple lesions + follicular lymphoblastoma	1
Lip — 1 lesion + skin — multiple lesions + larynx, SCE	1
Lip — 1 lesion + skin — multiple lesions + mouth, SCE	1
Lip — 1 lesion + skin — multiple lesions + prostate, ACA	1
Breasts, ACA, bilateral + other	12
Breasts, ACA, bilateral + stomach, ACA	2
Breasts, ACA, bilateral + uterine endometrium, ACA	2
Breasts, ACA, bilateral + colon, ACA	1
Breasts, ACA, bilateral + lymphosarcoma	1
Breasts, ACA, bilateral + ovary, adenoacanthoma	1
Breasts, ACA, bilateral + ovary, cystadenocarcinoma	1
Breasts, ACA, bilateral + skin, epithelioma	1
Breasts, ACA, bilateral + skin, multiple epitheliomas	1
Breasts, ACA, bilateral[1] + thyroid, ACA	1
Breasts, ACA, bilateral + colon, ACA + uterine endometrium, ACA	1
Ileum, carcinoids + other	4
Ileum, many carcinoids + lung, SCE	2
Ileum, many carcinoids + prostate, ACA	1
Ileum, many carcinoids + skin, multiple epitheliomas	1
Kidneys, hypernephromas + other	3
Kidneys, hypernephromas, bilateral + brain, oligodendroglioma	1

Table 6 (continued)

Site and type of malignant neoplasms	Cases
Kidneys, hypernephromas, bilateral + liposarcoma	1
Kidneys, hypernephromas, unilateral — 2 lesions + prostate, ACA	1
Bladder, kidney pelvis, ureter and urethra — epitheliomas + other	3
Bladder — 1 lesion + kidney pelvis — 1 lesion + colon, ACA	1
Bladder — 1 lesion + ureter — 1 lesion + esophagus, ACA	1
Kidney pelvis — 1 lesion + urethra + colon, ACA	1
Cervix, vagina, vulva and anus — SCE + other	3
Cervix + vagina + skin, multiple epitheliomas	1
Cervix + vulva + fibrosarcoma	1
Vagina + anus + skin, multiple epitheliomas	1
Lips, epitheliomas + other	2
Lips, epitheliomas — 2 lesions + stomach, ACA	1
Lips, epitheliomas — 2 lesions + fibrosarcoma + lung, SCE + parotid,	1
ACA + skin, multiple epitheliomas	
Mouth, SCE + other	2
Mouth, SCE — 2 lesions + skin, epithelioma	1
Mouth, SCE — 2 lesions + prostate, ACA	1
Stomach, ACA + other	2
Stomach — 2 lesions + pharynx, SCE	1
Stomach — 2 lesions + colon, ACA + kidney, hypernephroma	1
Mouth, tongue, pharynx, larynx and esophagus — SCE and lips, epitheliomas + other	2
Lip, epitheliomas + mouth, SCE + prostate, ACA	1
Pharynx, SCE + tongue, SCE + penis, SCE	1
Miscellaneous multicentric malignant neoplasms + other	6
Bladder, epitheliomas — 2 lesions + skin, multiple epitheliomas	1
Larynx, SCE — 2 lesions + skin, multiple epitheliomas	1
Tongue, SCE — 2 lesions + lung, ACA	1
Brain, astrocytoma + pituitary, pars nervosa, astrocytoma + uterus, ACA	1
Brain, multiple ependymomas + brain, astrocytoma	1
Testes, seminomas, bilateral + mouth, SCE + skin, epithelioma	1

[1] ACA = adenocarcinoma; SCE = squamous cell epithelioma.

Summary

Over the last half century, multiple primary malignant neoplasms have undergone a metamorphosis from being a rare medical curiosity to being a commonplace medical problem, one that is worthy of study not only because of its own intrinsic significance but also because it offers a new avenue of approach to the overall study of oncology.

By adhering to the criteria originally proposed by WARREN and GATES, we found that the presence of multiple primary malignant neoplasms had been proved pathologically in a total of 1,909 cases encountered at the Mayo Clinic during a 10-year period. Excluded from this number were the patients with multicentric epitheliomas

confined to the skin alone. These 1,909 patients represented an incidence of 5.1 %
among the 37,500 patients proved to have malignant disease by pathologic examination at this clinic during the same 10-year period. A more meaningful figure — the
number of patients with multiple primary malignant neoplasms of different tissues
of origin — was found to be 1,049 (2.8 %) of 37,580 patients.

When an individual has had two or more cancers of different tissues of origin,
it would seem likely that he has demonstrated a predisposition to malignant disease.
The physician should insist that such a patient have frequent and meticulous reexami-
nations so that any subsequent malignant disease may be discovered at an early and
curable stage.

All age groups from infancy to senescence were found to be vulnerable to
multiple cancers. No specific type of malignant neoplasm, neither common nor rare,
rendered any absolute immunity to the occurrence of another primary malignant
tumor.

References

BILLROTH, THEODOR: Die allgemeine chirurgische Pathologie und Therapie. 14 Aufl. Berlin:
   G. Reimer 1889, p. 908.
BLACK, HARRISON, and L. V. ACKERMAN: The importance of epidermoid carcinoma *in situ*
   in the histogenesis of carcinoma of the lung. Ann. Surg. **136**, 44 (1952).
COLLINS, W. T., and E. A. GALL: Gastric carcinoma: A multicentric lesion. Cancer (Philad.)
   5, 62 (1952).
DODGE, H. W., JR., H. M. KEITH, and M. J. CAMPAGNA: Intraspinal tumors in infants and
   children. J. int. Coll. Surg. **26**, 199 (1956).
EPSTEIN, ERVIN: Association of mucocutaneous and visceral cancers. Arch. Derm. Syph.
   (Chic.) **69**, 58 (1954).
HURT, R. E., and A. C. BRODERS: Multiple primary malignant neoplasms. J. Lab. clin. Med.
   18, 765 (1933).
LUND, C. C.: Second primary cancer in cases of cancer of the buccal mucosa: A mathematical
   study of susceptibility to cancer. New Engl. J. Med. **209**, 1144 (1933).
MacDONALD, ELEANOR J.: Occurrence of multiple primary cancers in a population of
   200,000. Acta Un. int. Cancr. **16**, 1702 (1960).
McGRATH, E. J., E. A. GALL, and D. P. KESSLER: Bronchogenic carcinoma, a product of
   multiple sites of origin. J. thorac. Surg. **24**, 271 (1952).
MERSHEIMER, W. L., ABRAHAM RINGEL, and HENRY EISENBERG: Some characteristics of mul-
   tiple primary cancers. Ann. N. Y. Acad. Sci. **114**, 896 (1964).
PELLER, SIGISMUND: Metachronous multiple malignancies in 5,876 cancer patients. Amer. J.
   Hyg. **34**, 1 (1941).
PHILLIPS, CHARLES: Multiple skin cancer: A statistical and pathologic study. Sth. med. J.
   (Bgham, Ala.) **35**, 583 (1942).
QUALHEIM, R. E., and E. A. GALL: Breast carcinoma with multiple sites of origin. Cancer
   (Philad.) **10**, 460 (1957).
SLAUGHTER, D. P.: The multiplicity of origin of malignant tumors: Collective review. Int.
   Abstr. Surg. **79**, 89 (1944). (*1*)
— Multicentric origin of intraoral carcinoma. Surg. **20**, 133 (1946). (*2*)
STALKER, L. E., R. B. PHILLIPS, and J. deJ. PEMBERTON: Multiple primary malignant lesions.
   Surg. Gynec. Obstet. **68**, 595 (1939).

WARREN, SHIELDS, and THEODORE EHRENREICH: Multiple primary malignant tumors and susceptibility to cancer. Cancer Res. 4, 554 (1944).

—, and OLIVE GATES: Multiple primary malignant tumors: A survey of the literature and a statistical study. Amer. J. Cancer. 16, 1358 (1932).

WATSON, T. A.: Incidence of multiple cancer. Cancer (Philad.) 6, 365 (1953).

WILLIAMS, MARJORIE J.: Extensive carcinoma in situ in the bronchial mucosa with two invasive bronchogenic carcinomas: Report of case. Cancer (Philad.) 5, 740 (1952).

WILLIS, R. A.: Further studies on the mode of origin of carcinomas of the skin. Cancer Res. 5, 469 (1945).

B. Multiple Primary Malignant Neoplasms of Different Tissues or Organs

1. Introductory Comments

When the inquiring physician encounters a patient with multiple malignant neoplasms of two or more different tissues of origin he will frequently succumb to the urge of speculation. He must wonder if serendipity has offered him in this patient the key to common etiologic influences inciting the two neoplasms, or perhaps to common factors of predisposition shared by the organs or tissues giving rise to these neoplasms. If the patient has received some form of therapy for an initial neoplasm, the physician may well question the possible role the therapeutic procedure might have had in inducing the subsequent neoplasm. Perhaps patients with two distinct types of cancer may show more distinct hereditary patterns than have been demonstrable to date in patients with single cancers. When one is studying a group of patients with multiple primary cancers, the urge to such speculation becomes almost irresistible.

Not only does the literature suggest that the existence of one malignant neoplasm implies increased susceptibility to the development of a second lesion, but it also has suggested that a malignant lesion in one organ may imply increased susceptibility of another organ to a malignant neoplasm, particularly another organ in the same or in an associated system. When a patient presents with two primary malignant neoplasms in each of two organs of the same system, it is tempting for the physician to state that this patient has demonstrated either susceptibility of the entire system to neoplastic disease or the presence of a carcinogenic influence to which the particular organ system is susceptible. HURT and BRODERS were so impressed with this tendency that after studying 71 cases of multiple primary cancers they reached the following categorical conclusion: "... if a malignant neoplasm develops in one organ of a system, another primary malignant neoplasm is more likely to develop in that organ or in an organ of the same system."

In the previous section we pointed out the almost insurmountable difficulty of establishing the hypothesis that the existence of any malignant neoplasm implies an increased susceptibility to the future development of malignant disease. The statistical problems are compounded if an attempt is made to prove that a specific neoplasm implies an increased susceptibility to another specific neoplasm, or to a designated group of specific neoplasms. Some authors have tried to circumvent this problem by comparing the relative frequency of certain combinations of neoplasms among all patients with multiple cancers. Here again many hidden sources of error could cause gross distortion of the facts presented. The mean ages of patients at the time of occurrence of each specific neoplasm vary over a wide range, as do the survival rates of the patients with each specific neoplasm; both of these factors have a great influence on the relative frequency with which a specific second cancer would be observed.

Many of the conclusions stated in the literature regarding patterns of occurrence of multiple primary cancers of different tissues of origin are highly questionable since the statistical methods used to reach these conclusions have been of doubtful validity. Nevertheless, and in spite of the obstacles discussed above, there have been a few very significant and meaningful observations derived from studies of this kind, particularly with regard to the role of therapeutic procedures in the induction of second cancers. These will be discussed in the following pages.

In this section four major points will be discussed: (1) the occurrence of multiple cancers within the same or related organ systems, (2) second primary cancers induced by treatment of an initial malignant neoplasm, (3) hereditary influences in patients with multiple primary malignant neoplasms of different tissues of origin, and (4) blood groups and multiple primary cancers. In addition, because of special interest evidenced in the literature, detailed discussions will be given regarding the association of other primary malignant neoplasms with leukemias and lymphomas, with the carcinoid tumor, and with primary lung cancers.

Reference

Hurt, H. H., and A. C. Broders: Multiple primary malignant neoplasms. J. Lab. clin. Med. **18**, 765 (1933).

2. Occurrence of Multiple Cancers Within the Same or Related Organ Systems

a) Multiple Cancers Involving the Female Genitalia and Breasts

Most of the literature concerned with the tendency of multiple cancers to develop in the same or in related organ systems is based on the purported tendency in women who have primary neoplasms of the breast or female genitalia to develop second primary cancer in these same estrogen-influenced organs. In 1931 Taylor reported 18 cases of primary cancer of the breast associated with one or more other primary cancers. He found that in 55 % of his cases the associated cancer was in the genital tract. He was most impressed with the relative preponderance of associated adenocarcinomas of the uterus in his series (four cases), and he implied that there was a connection between the carcinoma of the breast and the adenocarcinoma of the uterus. In 1948 Pierce and Slaughter reported 3 cases of pelvic carcinoma among 63 cases of cancer of the breast. To them this finding indicated a tendency to the development of cancer in the two systems, so that some common etiologic factor might well be indicated. Later in the same year, Speert reported that of 622 patients with carcinoma of the cervix, only 5 (0.8 %) had cancer of the breast, whereas of 255 patients with carcinoma of the uterus, 6 (2.4 %) had cancer of the breast. He suggested that there was a common estrogenic stimulus for both endometrial and mammary neoplasms. Huber also has written extensively about this problem. He found that of 75 extragenital carcinomas occurring with genital carcinoma, 30 (40.0 %) were carcinomas of the breast. He stated that the breasts were connected functionally with the formation of tumors of the uterus, ovaries, and oviducts.

That abnormal estrogenic stimulation of the breasts and female genitalia may incite neoplastic growth is an appealing hypothesis since estrogen is a normal stimulus of growth of these organs. Indeed, this thesis has proved true in some experimental animals. An equally appealing corollary to this theory is that when one estrogen-sensitive organ has given rise to a cancer, other estrogen-sensitive organs are more likely to fall under the same carcinogenic spell. However, it seems highly questionable whether this proposal has been established as fact.

In Table 7 the percentage distribution found in this study of the specific second primary malignant neoplasms occurring in women with cancers of the breast and genitalia is compared with that found in women with cancer of the large bowel. Second cancers of the breast were represented in essentially the same proportion in patients with cancer of the large bowel (29 %) as they were in patients with cancer of the genitalia (27 and 34 %). Likewise, it can be seen that patients with carcinoma of the breast did not show a significant greater proportion of second cancers of the female genitalia when compared with patients with carcinoma of the colon.

Table 7. *Comparative Frequency of Occurrence of Specific Second Primary Malignant Neoplasms in Women With Primary Cancers of the Colon, Breast, and Genitalia*

| Primary cancer Site of origin | Cases | Site of origin of second primary cancers, percentage distribution | | | | | |
		Colon	Breast	Cervix	Uterus	Ovary	All others
Colon	105	...	29	7	14	7	43
Breast	148	20	...	7	18	10	43
Cervix	52	8	27	...	6	11	48
Uterus	80	14	34	6	...	13	33
Ovary	48	13	27	13	19	...	28

In patients with cancers of the breast, the ratio of a second independent cancer of the cervix to a second cancer of the uterus (7 to 18) seems disproportionate to the expected ratio in the general population. Observation of a similar disproportion led TAYLOR to suggest the possibility of a connection between development of cancers of the breast and the appearance of adenocarcinomas of the uterus. In Table 7, however, essentially the same disproportion (7 to 14) will be noted in the second cancers of patients with carcinoma of the colon. These disproportions probably are explained most easily by the fact that the average age at occurrence of carcinoma of the cervix is several years younger than the average age at occurrence of most other types of malignant neoplasms. Many of these patients with carcinoma of the cervix die before they reach the age when they presumably would be most susceptible to other malignant disease. Of 823 patients with proved carcinoma of the cervix seen during the period of this study, only 52 (6.3 %) had second primary lesions, whereas of 807 patients with carcinoma of the uterus, 80 (9.9 %) had second primary neoplasms. Thus it is evident that a patient with carcinoma of the cervix has a lower incidence of all second malignant neoplasms; this is not specific for the breast.

None of the studies cited above nor, indeed, our own figures offer any reliable information regarding the association of multiple cancers of the female genitalia and breasts, because the statistical methods employed are obviously invalid. Recently, this problem has been approached by Bailar with more sophisticated statistical methodology. He compared the incidence of second cancers in women who had primary malignant neoplasms of the cervix and uterus with that in women of the general population, utilizing material submitted to the Connecticut Cancer Case Registry. He expressed his data in terms of incidence per person-years of exposure, and also calculated his data individually for given patient age groups. His data showed that in patients with carcinoma of the cervix the observed incidence of cancers of the rectum, lung, oral cavity, bladder, and skin was greater than the expected incidence. The observed incidence of breast cancer was equal to that expected, and the observed incidence of cancer of the digestive organs, other than the large bowel, was less than that expected. Patients with carcinoma of the uterus had a greater than expected incidence of carcinoma of the oral cavity, colon and rectum, breast, and skin. Actually, the increased incidence of second cancers of the colon was much more impressive than second cancers of the breast. Whereas these observations are of interest, they are, unfortunately, of no significance. While the statistical methods employed by BAILAR were much superior to those of previous studies, his clinical material was decidedly inferior to the point of being unreliable. The following major objections to the sources of data used in BAILAR's study must be raised:

1. In a number of cases, the diagnosis of cancer was made on purely clinical grounds without any surgical, autopsy, or histologic confirmation.

2. A patient was accepted as having a second primary cancer when it was so stated by the "attending physician" regardless of his qualifications or of the particular criteria he may have used to reach this conclusion.

3. When pathologic material was obtained from each neoplasm, this material was not reviewed to confirm that the second lesions were, indeed, primary cancers rather than metastasis or recurrence of the initial malignant neoplasm.

The great source of error introduced by the lack of proper confirmation of data was made manifest when the pathologic material from a small segment of the patient group, namely those with cancers of the bladder subsequent to cervical or uterine cancers, was reviewed by a skilled pathologist. Almost half of the reported cases were discarded. If these cases had been included, the frequency of second cancers primary to the bladder in this series would have been increased by 67%. When such a striking magnitude of error can be uncovered by careful case study, the validity of all of the other cases, which were not so studied, must be seriously questioned and any conclusions drawn from these cases nullified.

We may conclude then that neither this study nor the literature offers any convincing evidence that malignant disease in an estrogen-sensitive organ increases the probality of carcinogenesis in other estrogen-sensitive organs. One possible and rare exception to this statement may be the occurrence of endometrial carcinoma in women with functioning ovarian neoplasms, where first endometrial hyperplasia and then uterine cancer is presumed to be induced by prolonged and excessive estrogen stimulation.

b) Coexistence of Epithelial Carcinoma of the Bladder and Adenocarcinoma of the Prostate

In their study of multiple cancers reported to the Connecticut Cancer Case Registry, MERSHEIMER and associates noted the frequent coexistence of carcinomas of the bladder and the prostate. They cited this as evidence for a systemic tendency to cancer of the genitourinary tract.

In this study as well, the combination of epitheliomas of the bladder and adenocarcinomas of the prostate was a frequent observation, second in frequency only to the combination of two much more common neoplasms — skin cancer and colonic cancer. It is certainly true that the combined occurrence of these two genitourinary cancers would seem more common than chance alone would allow. Before one accepts this as evidence for a systemic tendency to cancer, however, the possibility of some artifact in case finding must be considered. Both carcinoma of the prostate and low-grade papillary carcinomas of the bladder frequently exist in clinically benign forms and may commonly be diagnosed as "incidental findings" during surgery for other reasons or at autopsy. Papillary bladder cancers may be found incidentally during surgery for prostatic carcinoma, and prostatic cancers may be found incidentally during transurethral resections performed in the process of treating papillary bladder carcinomas. Many of the coexistent bladder and prostate cancers in this study were diagnosed in this manner. In 68 % of the patients with the combination of bladder and prostatic carcinomas in this series, the neoplasms had been diagnosed simultaneously, whereas only 38 % of all patients with multiple cancers of different tissues of origin had simultaneously occurring lesions.

In view of the above considerations, it would seem that more substantial evidence must be presented before the frequent reporting of coincident bladder and prostate carcinomas can be accepted as indicating a systemic tendency to carcinogenesis rather than an artifact related to diagnostic and case-finding procedures.

References

BAILAR, J. C., III: The incidence of independent tumors among uterine cancer patients. Cancer (Philad.) 16, 842 (1963).

HUBER, HERBERT: Genitalkarzinom und Mammakarzinom als Multiplizitätstumoren. Strahlentherapie 92, 130 (1953).

MERSHEIMER, W. L., A. RINGEL, and H. EISENBERG: Some characteristics of multiple primary cancers. Ann. N. Y. Acad. Sci. 114, 896 (1964).

PIERCE, VIRGINIA K., and D. P. SLAUGHTER: The association of breast and pelvic disease. Cancer (Philad.) 1, 468 (1948).

SPEERT, HAROLD: Corpus cancer. Clinical, pathological and etiological aspects. Cancer (Philad.) 1, 584 (1948).

TAYLOR, H. C.: The coincidence of primary breast and uterine cancer. Amer. J. Cancer. 15, 277 (1931).

3. Second Primary Cancers Induced by Treatment of an Initial Malignant Neoplasm

Modern medical, surgical, and roentgenologic means of treating malignant disease have in common the production of significant changes in body physiology. The effectiveness of medical and roentgenologic treatment especially is in a large measure directly proportional to the change in physiology produced. Unfortunately, these therapeutic procedures produce physiologic changes that are not confined to the neoplasm being attacked; they also may produce changes in adjacent tissues, as well as in more remote tissues. The possibility must be recognized that by these changes the therapeutic means which will retard malignant disease in one tissue may be carcinogenic to another tissue. The carcinogenic effects of ionizing radiation seem well established, and carcinogenic effects may well be suspected for the hormonal and tissue toxic agents used at present in oncologic therapy.

a) Therapeutic Ionizing Radiation

Radiation therapy as a curative rather than a palliative measure probably is employed most frequently for women with carcinoma of the cervix. Since many of these patients survive for long periods of time after treatment, the possibility that other uterine malignant disease may be induced by the radiation therapy is of considerable importance. The possible role of irradiation as a cause of cancer of the uterine fundus was studied by SPEERT and PEIGHTAL and by SCHEFFEY. The former authors found that about 8 % of women with cancer of the fundus in their series had had previous irradiation of the fundus, and they suggested that irradiation may have a carcinogenic effect on the uterine fundus. In SCHEFFEY's series 10 % of the women with cancer of the fundus had had previous irradiation of the fundus. He concluded that factors other than irradiation were responsible for the development of the uterine cancers. With such opposing statements, it must be suspected that the evidence for a carcinogenic effect of irradiation on the uterine fundus is at best equivocal.

Four patients in our series had both squamous cell carcinomas of the cervix and adenocarcinomas of the uterine fundus. Two of these patients had had radiation treatment for carcinoma of the cervix before the carcinoma of the fundus developed. In both of the other patients the two lesions were diagnosed simultaneously. Considering the fact that 832 cases of carcinoma of the cervix and 813 cases of carcinoma of the uterine fundus were diagnosed at the Mayo Clinic during the period covered by this study, it is difficult to assign much significance to the occurrence of two cases in which an irradiation-treated carcinoma of the cervix preceded an adenocarcinoma of the fundus. In a more detailed presentation of these two cases, FRICKE stated that since such occurrences are so rare, other unknown factors must operate with the possible carcinogenic effect of irradiation.

In 1953 DELARUE and associates reported a case of carcinoma of the thyroid treated with successive large doses of radioactive iodine (^{131}I). Significant reduction in the size of metastatic lesions and amelioration of symptoms resulted. Directly following this reatment, however, pancytopenia developed; and within 2 years, frank acute myelogenous leukemia, which later caused the patient's death, was diagnosed.

Subsequently, 10 additional cases of leukemia occurring subsequent to ^{131}I therapy of thyroid carcinoma have appeared in the literature (Table 8). In all cases, the leukemia was myelogenous and usually of the acute or subacute type. The average interval from onset of therapy to diagnosis of leukemia was approximately $3^{1}/_{2}$ years. Most patients had had repeated courses of ^{131}I therapy during this period. In many patients the diagnosis of frank leukemia was preceded, as in the case of DELARUE, by a period of pancytopenia. Evidence that the leukemia in these patients is more than just chance occurrence is provided by the impressive incidence of acute myelogenous leukemia in patients treated with ^{131}I for thyroid cancer: 4 of 141 cases in the series of POCHIN and 2 of 16 cases in the series of SEIDLIN and associates.

Table 8. *Cases of Leukemia Following [131]I Therapy of Thyroid Carcinoma*

Author	Dose of ^{131}I MC	Interval: onset of ^{131}I therapy to diagnosis of leukemia (months)	Type of leukemia
DELARUE et al.	324[1]	34	Acute myelogenous
BLOM et al.	261[1]	9	Acute myelogenous
SEIDLIN et al.	1,455	54[2]	Acute myelogenous
SEIDLIN et al.	1,730	60[2]	Acute myelogenous
JELLIFFE and JONES	400	24	Acute myelogenous
OZARDA et al.	347	40	Chronic myelogenous
POCHIN	1,130	41	Acute myelogenous
POCHIN	1,280	36	Acute myelogenous
POCHIN	1,430	32	Acute myelogenous
POCHIN	1,715	47	Acute myelogenous
LEWALLEN and GODWIN	805	44	Acute myelogenous

[1] Patient also received external radiation to the neck.
[2] Approximate time period.

A very strong chain of circumstantial evidence has been forged which indicates that massive doses of radioisotopes do have a leukemogenic effect.

Evidence for a leukemogenic effect of external radiation, as used in cancer therapy, is far less impressive than that for systemically administered radioisotopes. Cases of leukemia occurring subsequent to radiation therapy for breast or cervical carcinoma have appeared sporadically in the literature (see below), but the number of such cases is not imposing when viewed in the light of the many thousands of patients so treated. SIMON and associates collected data regarding 71,582 women treated with radiation therapy for carcinoma of the cervix. Leukemia developed in only 16 of this group after therapy. These cases represented an incidence of 115 per million person years. SIMON and associates stated that this incidence was essentially the expected incidence of leukemia in women of similar age in the United States and Great Britain. They concluded that radiation therapy for carcinoma of the cervix does not induce an increase in the incidence of leukemia among the survivors.

b) The Stewart-Treves Syndrome

In 1948 the informed curiosity of STEWART and TREVES brought to light a theretofore unrecognized phenomenon — the predilection of lymphangiosarcomas (or angiosarcomas) to form in regions of chronic lymph stasis.

All of the six cases initially reported by these authors were cases of lymphangiosarcoma developing at the site of lymphedema after radical excision of cancers of the breast. In subsequent reports this combination has been appropriately designated as the Stewart-Treves syndrome. In 1963, CHU and TREVES gathered an additional 39 such cases from the literature, to which they added 4 of their own. Other cases appearing prior to this writing (BLOCK et al.; BOSS and URKA; CONTE and RELLA; CUKIER;

DE JAGER; DELARUE; GIANNARDI et al.; HUME et al.; KHODADADEH et al.; OOTA and BABA; LAFFARGUE et al.; MARTIN and VILAIN; MARTORELL; OGILVY et al.; PATARO and ACRICH; RENÉ et al.; RYDELL et al.; SALM; STERNBY; STERNBY et al.; TASWELL et al.; TENTSCHOV et al.; U. S. Naval Medical School; VANDAELE et al.; and WILSON) have brought the total of reported cases to 89. We have included one such case in this study.

The pathogenetic mechanism underlying this interesting phenomenon has not been delineated clearly as yet. STEWART and TREVES stated that no other cases of lymphangiosarcoma occurring in lymphedema of any cause had been reported in the literature. Since the lymphangiosarcomas in all of their cases occurred at the site of postmastectomy lymphedema, they proposed that chronic lymph stasis in itself is not an adequate stimulus. They theorized that the coexistence of cancer of the breast and lymphangiosarcoma implied that these patients had some type of systemic carcinogen in addition to lymph stasis.

The report of McCONNELL and HASLAM considerably weakened this thesis, for they found nine cases in the literature, in both men and women, in which angiosarcomas developed in lymphedematous extremities in the absence of any previous malignant disease. Five additional similar cases have subsequently been reported (DE JAGER, TASWELL et al., and VANDAELE et al.). Chronic lymph stasis alone, therefore, may be sufficient stimulus to initiate sarcomatous change in the susceptible patient. There is no acceptable evidence that mammary cancer itself in any way predisposes the patient to the development of lymphangiosarcoma, or that the coexistence of mammary cancer and lymphangiosarcoma implies any systemic carcinogenic influence.

c) Carcinoma of the Male Breast Developing during Estrogen Therapy for Carcinoma of the Prostate

Since estrogen has been shown to be an effective carcinogenic agent in some experimental animals, it has been hypothesized that this hormone may have a carcinogenic influence on the estrogen-sensitive human tissues. Studies of this relationship in malignant neoplasms of the human female genitalia or breast have not brought forth any convincing confirmatory evidence. Strong verification for this hypothesis, however, could be afforded if it could be demonstrated that cancer of the breast developed in a significant number of males while they were under treatment with large doses of estrogenlike substances for carcinoma of the prostate.

Presumably with this objective in mind, many case reports have appeared in the literature of malignant lesions of the breast in males receiving hormonal therapy for carcinoma of the prostate. BENSON reviewed these reports. Several authors were so impressed with the danger of inducing breast cancer that they cautioned the physician to examine the breast carefully and frequently during the period of hormonal therapy.

An analysis of the cases in the literature reveals that, in the vast majority, the lesions of both the prostate and the breast were highly anaplastic adenocarcinomas, and the lesion in the breast quite probably was metastatic. For only one case, that of JAKOBSEN, does there seem to be clear evidence that the lesion in the breast was primary to that tissue and not metastatic from a single primary prostatic neoplasm.

Two patients seen at the Mayo Clinic during the period of this study had malignant lesions involving both breast and prostate; one patient had had estrogen therapy, the other had not. In each case, both lesions were highly anaplastic adeno-carcinomas, and they were indistinguishable under the microscope. Of 1,720 patients with pathologically proved carcinoma of the prostate seen at the Mayo Clinic during the 10 years covered by this study, none had primary cancer of the breast.

References

BENSON, W. R.: Carcinoma of the prostate with metastases to breasts and testis: Critical review of the literature and report of a case. Cancer (Philad.) 10, 1235 (1957).

BLOCK, M. A., J. L. FLEMING, and J. R. GISH: Lymphangiosarcoma occurring in postmastectomy lymphedema. Henry Ford Hosp. Bull. 4, 63 (1956).

BLOM, P. S., A. QUERIDO, and C. H. W. LEEKSMA: Acute leukaemia following x-ray and radioiodine treatment of thyroid carcinoma. Brit. J. Radiol. 28, 165 (1955).

BOSS, J. H., and J. URKA: Stewart-Treves syndrome: Angiosarcoma in postmastectomy lymphedema associated with disseminated vascular lesions. Amer. J. Surg. 101, 248 (1961).

CHU, FLORENCE C. H., and NORMAN TREVES: The value of radiation therapy in postmast-ectomy lymphangiosarcoma. Amer. J. Roentgen. 89, 64 (1963).

CONTE, A. J., and A. J. RELLA: Angiosarcoma in lymphedema following mastectomy. N. Y. med. J. 62, 3966 (1962).

CUKIER, J.: Lymphangio-sarcomes développés sur gros bras après amputation du sein pour cancer. Ann. Chir. 14, 833 (1960).

DE JAGER, H.: Secundair lymfangiosarcoom. Ned. T. Geneesk. 107, 1344 (1963).

DELARUE, J.: Les résidives-métastases brachiales des cancers due sein (et les prétendus lymphangiosarcomes des bras lymphoedémateux après mammectomie). Mém. Acad. Chir. 88, 98 (1962).

—, M. TUBIANA et J. DUTREIX: Cancer de la thyroïde traité par l'iode radiactif: Terminaison par une leucémie aiguë après une amélioration importante. Bull. Ass. franç. Cancer 40, 263 (1953).

FRICKE, R. E.: Two unusual cases of pelvic cancer. J. Amer. Geriat. Soc. 2, 324 (1954).

GIANNARDI, G. F., G. PELÙ e G. ZAMPI: Il quardo clinoco e le basi istopatologiche della cosidetta sindrome di Stewart e Treves. Arch. De Vecchi Anat. pat. 34, 361 (1960).

HUME, H. A., W. H. ERB, and L. W. STEVENS: Lymphangiosarcoma following radical mastectomy. Surg. Gynec. Obstet. 116, 117 (1963).

JAKOBSEN, A. H. I.: Bilateral mammary carcinoma in the male following stilboestrol therapy. Acta path. microbiol. scand. 31, 61 (1952).

JELLIFFE, A. M., and K. M. JONES: Leukaemia after I131 therapy for thyroid cancer. Clin. Radiol. 11, 134 (1960).

KHODADADEH, MANUCHEHR, RICHARD JOHNSON, and G. W. ZEIDERS: Lymphangiosarcoma arising from postmastectomy lymphedema. J. Amer. med. Ass. 186, 1097 (1963).

LAFFARGUE, P., F. PINET, and R. LE GO: Syndrome de Stewart et Treves (métastases épithéliomateuses ou angiosarcome dans les gros bras compliquant la mammectomie). Presse méd. 68, 1506 (1960).

LEWALLEN, C. G., and J. T. GODWIN: Acute myelogenous leukemia complicating radioactive iodine therapy of thyroid cancer. Amer. J. Roentgen. 89, 610 (1963).

MARTIN, E., and R. VILAIN: Discussion anatomique sur un ces de syndrome de Stewart-Trèves. Arch. Anat. path. 8, 246 (1960).

MARTORELL, F.: Linfangiosarcoma postmastectomia. Angiologia. 16, 208 (1964).

McCONNELL, E. M., and P. HASLAM: Angiosarcoma in postmastectomy lymphoedema: A report of 5 cases and a review of the literature. Brit. J. Surg. 46, 322 (1959).

OGILVY, W. L., R. H. FRANKLIN, and IAN AIRD: Angioblastic sarcoma in post-mastectomy lymphoedema. Canad. J. Surg. 2, 195 (1959).

OOTA, KUNIO, and TSUNEO BABA: A case of postmastectomy lymphangiosarcoma. Gann 47, 748 (1956).

OZARDA, AHSEN, UMIT ERGIN, and M. A. BENDER: Chronic myelogenous leukemia following
    I[131] therapy for metastatic thyroid carcinoma: Report of a case and some considerations
    on the etiologic factors. Amer. J. Roentgen. 85, 914 (1961).

PATARO, V. F., and M. W. ACRICH: Angiosarcoma postmastectomia: Síndrome de Stewart-
    Treves. Pren. méd. argent. 51, 802 (1964).

POCHIN, E. E.: The Occurrence of Leukaemia Following Radioiodine Therapy. In Pitt-
    Rivers, Rosalind: Advances in Thyroid Research: Transactions of the Fourth International
    Goitre Conference, London, July, 1960. New York: Pergamon Press 1961, pp. 392—397.

RENÉ, L., M. BOLGERT, M. LE SOURD, J. TABERNAT et R. POISSON: Un cas de syndrome de
    Stewart-Treves. Bull. Soc. franç. Derm. Syph. 70, 9 (1963).

RYDELL, J. R., W. K. JENNINGS, and E. T. SMITH: Postmastectomy lymphedema. Calif. Med.
    89, 390 (1958).

SALM, R.: The nature of the so-called postmastectomy lymphangiosarcoma. J. Path. Bact. 85,
    445 (1963).

SCHEFFEY, L. C.: Malignancy subsequent to irradiation of the uterus for benign conditions.
    Amer. J. Obstet. Gynec. 44, 925 (1942).

SEIDLIN, S. M., EDWARD SIEGEL, S. MELAMED, and A. A. YALOW: Occurrence of myeloid
    leukemia in patients with metastatic thyroid carcinoma following prolonged massive
    radioiodine therapy. Bull. N. Y. Acad. Med. 31, 410 (1955).

SIMON, NORMAN, MARSHALL BRUCER, and RAYMOND HAYES: Radiation and leukemia in
    carcinoma of the cervix. Radiology 74, 905 (1960).

SPEERT, HAROLD, and T. C. PEIGHTAL: Malignant tumors of the uterine fundus subsequent
    to irradiation for benign pelvic conditions. Amer. J. Obstet. Gynec. 57, 261 (1949).

STERNBY, N. H.: Lympfangiosarkom efter mastektomi. (Abstr.) Nord. med. 61, 291 (1959).

—, I. GYNNING, and K. E. HOGEMAN: Postmastectomy angiosarcoma. Acta chir. scand. 121,
    420 (1961).

STEWART, F. W., and W. TREVES: Lymphangiosarcoma in postmastectomy lymphedema:
    A report of six cases in elephantiasis chirurgica. Cancer (Philad.) 1, 64 (1948).

TASWELL, H. F., E. H. SOULE, and M. B. COVENTRY: Lymphangiosarcoma arising in chronic
    lymphedematous extremities. J. Bone Jt Surg. 44-A, 277 (1962).

TENTSCHOV, G., V. ANDREEV, R. RAITSCHEV, and B. KRISTEV: Lymphangiosarkom bei Lymph-
    ödem nach Ablatio Mammae (Stewart-Treves-Syndrom). Hautarzt. 12, 399 (1961).

United States Naval Medical School of the National Medical Center: Color Atlas of
    Pathology. Philadelphia: J. B. Lippincott Company 1950, vol. 1, p. 243.

VANDAELE, R., W. V. CRAEYNEST, E. HAVEN, and A. DUPONT: Lymphangiosarcome sur
    lymphoedème primitif du bras. Bull. Soc. franç. Derm. Syph. 70, 722 (1963).

WILSON, ROGER: Lymphangiosarcoma in the post-mastectomy lymphedematous arm. Canad.
    J. Surg. 5, 208 (1962).

4. Hereditary Influences in Patients with Multiple Primary Malignant Neoplasms

"Nothing about cancer is more generally accepted than its hereditary nature, and nothing is less satisfactorily proved" (EWING).

Although hereditary factors are evident in the genesis of malignant neoplasms in some experimental animals, there is little factual information to support the concept that such factors have an influence on neoplasia in man. The difficulties encountered in attempting any large-scale, accurate, and well-controlled study in this regard seem almost insurmountable.

It may be conjectured that hereditary influence in malignant disease may be brought out in bolder relief by a study of patients who have had two or more independent primary malignant neoplasms. The literature concerned with multiple primary cancers is liberally sprinkled with percentage figures on the family history of malignant disease as given by the patients included in the series reported. The incidences given have varied from 14% of the patients in the series of TULLIS to 50% in the series of WELCH. Figures of this kind have little comparative value since they probably reflect to a large extent the diligence of the historians and the memory and knowledge of the patients.

The study to be reported here suffers from all the limitations and inaccuracies of any retrospective study based on second-hand information obtained by reviewing medical histories. It is hoped that these limitations may be offset in some measure by the use of a large group of patients and by the use of appropriate control groups. Here again, however, volume alone does not ensure the validity of conclusions, and even the most carefully chosen control group is subject to question when one is dealing with such a nebulous entity as hereditary influence in malignant disease.

The family histories obtained in the admission interviews of 2,346 patients were studied, and data regarding 6,681 family members were recorded. To ensure reasonable historical accuracy and the most direct applicability to the patient, only information regarding the immediate family was used — that is, concerning parents, siblings, and children. Data regarding a member of the family were recorded only if the patient had stated the present age or age at death of the member of the family. A member of the family was recorded as having malignant disease only if an unequivocal statement was made confirming the presence of cancer; vague terms such as "tumor" were not accepted.

The patients and the corresponding members of their families were gathered into three groups: Group I consisted of 2,266 members of the families of 782 patients who had multiple primary malignant neoplasms of different tissues of origin confirmed pathologically at the Mayo Clinic from 1944 through 1953. Patients with multicentric cancers alone were not included. Group II consisted of 2,234 members of the families of 782 patients each of whom had a single malignant neoplasm that was confirmed by pathologic examination at the Mayo Clinic from 1944 through 1953. The specific types of malignant neoplasms were chosen so that they would have proportionately the same representation as those of the patients in group I. The sex ratio was the same as that of the patients in group I. The average age and the age distribution at the time of diagnosis of the single malignant neoplasm were the same as those in group I at the time of diagnosis of multiple malignant neoplasms. Group III consisted of 2,181 members of the families of 782 patients who were seen at this clinic from 1944 through 1953. They did not give any history of previous malignant disease and on examination showed no evidence of malignant disease. The sex ratio, average age, and age distribution were the same as those for groups I and II.

The results of this study are summarized graphically in Fig. 2. When the occurrence rate of malignant disease was determined for all family members, that of members of the families of patients with single malignant neoplasms (group II) did not differ significantly from that of the families of patients without malignant disease (group III). Members of the families of patients with multiple cancers, on the other hand, showed a 26% increase in the incidence of malignant disease over that seen in members of the families of patients without malignant disease.

A much more striking difference was evidenced when the occurrence rate of malignant disease in members of the families before the age of 50 years was determined. Here members of the families of the patients with single cancers showed a

37 % increase, and members of the families of the patients with multiple cancers showed a 149 % increase over the incidence seen in the families of patients with no evidence of malignant disease.

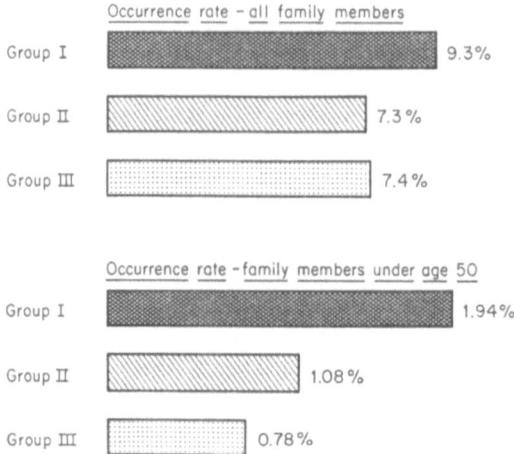

Fig. 2. Comparative occurrence rates of malignant disease in members of the families of patients with multiple primary malignant neoplasms (group I), patients with single malignant neoplasms (group II), and patients with no evidence of malignant disease (group III)

The members of the families of the patients with multiple primary malignant neoplasms had a somewhat higher overall occurrence rate of malignant disease, with a more definitely increased occurrence rate of malignant disease in the younger age groups. In view of the limitations of this study, however, it would be presumptuous to assign any statistical significance to these figures or to purport that they are representative of all patients with single and multiple malignant neoplasms. It may only be hoped that these results may provide some guidelines to more sophisticated prospective studies in the future.

References

EWING, JAMES: Neoplastic diseases, Ed. 2. Philadelphia: W. B. Saunders Company 1922, p. 105.

TULLIS, J. L.: Multiple primary malignant lesions. J. Lab. clin. Med. 27, 588 (1942).

WELCH, J. W.: Multiple primary malignant lesions. J. Kans. med. Soc. 55, 314 (1954).

5. Blood Groups and Multiple Primary Malignant Neoplasms

A fad in recent medical literature has been the attempt to associate blood groups with various disease states. In respect to malignant neoplasms, with the possible exception of gastric carcinoma, these studies have met with negative or equivocal results. In 1963, FADHLI and DOMINGUEZ reviewed a small group of patients with multiple primary malignant neoplasms and reported a statistically significant excess of blood group A. They suggested a predisposition to the development of a second cancer in patients with one cancer that was at least in part associated with the ABO system, and further, that in the type A individual a second cancer is more likely to develop. They made a clarion call for routine determination of the blood group of every patient in whom a diagnosis of cancer has been established. These conclusions, however, have subsequently been somewhat dampened by the cold water of a conflicting study. TSUKADA and associates reported a blood-group study of 310 patients with multiple primary malignant neoplasms. They did not find a significant increase in blood group A among their multiple-cancer patients, nor did they find an increase in blood group A in any specific combination of multiple cancers. With the hope of perhaps resolving this conflict, an analysis was made of the patients with multiple primary malignant neoplasms in this study.

ABO blood groups were recorded for 731 of our patients with multiple cancers of different tissues of origin and for 396 of those with the most common types of multicentric cancers. Two groups of Mayo Clinic patients were used as controls. The first group consisted of 1,004 patients in whom a single malignant neoplasm had been diagnosed during the 10-year period of this study. Specific types of tumors in these patients were represented in similar proportion as those in the patients with multiple cancers. The second control group was composed of Mayo Clinic blood group data compiled by MAGATH and BERKSON. This data involved 100,000 unselected Mayo Clinic patients in whom blood groups were obtained during the period 1950 to 1959, inclusive. A third group of control data was gathered from the literature (ALBRITTON and HERVEY et al.).

In Table 9 it can be seen that there was no difference of consequence in the representation of ABO blood groups and Rh(D) blood groups when patients with

Table 9. *Blood Groups in Patients With Multiple Cancers of Different Tissues of Origin, Patients With Single Cancers, and Control Populations*

Blood group	Multiple cancers, % of 731 patients	Single cancers, % of 1,004	Mayo Clinic[1], % of 100,000	Rochester, N.Y.,[2] % of 23,787	Detroit, Mich.,[2] % of 5,728	Columbus, Ohio,[2] % of 5,869	Massachusetts,[2] % of 23,322	Region unspecified,[3] % of 20,000
0	45.4	44.1	43.0	44.4	41.8	44.0	46.3	45.0
A	40.4	39.7	42.0	41.8	41.0	43.2	39.7	41.0
B	10.1	10.9	11.0	10.0	11.9	9.2	10.6	10.0
AB	4.1	5.3	4.0	3.8	5.2	3.6	3.4	4.0
	(% of 600)	(% of 869)	(% of 7,260)[4]					
Rh pos.	85.5	83.5	84.3					
Rh neg.	14.5	16.5	15.7					

[1] MAGATH and BERKSON   [2] HERVEY et al.   [3] ALBRITTON   [4] TASWELL

Table 10. *Blood Groups in Patients With Multicentric Cancers and Control Populations*

Blood groups	Multicentric, colon and rectum, % of 197 patients	Multicentric, urinary tract, % of 60	Multicentric, upper aerodigestive tract,[1] % of 48	Bilateral breast, % of 91	Control groups,[2] % (range)		
0	43.1	46.7	45.8	49.5	41.8	to	46.3
A	42.2	35.0	35.4	39.5	39.7	to	43.2
B	11.7	15.0	14.6	6.6	9.2	to	11.9
AB	3.0	3.3	4.2	5.5	3.4	to	5.2

[1] Lips, oral cavity, larynx, pharynx, and esophagus.   [2] See Table 9.

multiple cancers of different tissues of origin were compared with patients who had single cancers, with a large overall group of Mayo Clinic patients, or with several control groups from different regions of the United States. Comparable results were also obtained with regard to ABO blood groups in the major types of multicentric cancers (Table 10). In no instance did the proportionate representation of any blood group show a statistically significant difference from the range of control values. Specifically, no higher frequency of blood group A was noted.

These results offer strong support to the conclusions of TSUKADA and associates. We cannot support the suggestion of FADHLI and DOMINGUEZ that a predisposition to second cancers is associated with the ABO system or that in the type A individual a second cancer is more likely to develop. We see no need for the routine determination of blood groups in cancer patients unless a blood transfusion is contemplated.

References

ALBRITTON, E. C.: Standard values in blood. Philadelphia: W. B. Saunders Company 1952, p. 26.

FADHLI, H. A., and R. DOMINGUEZ: ABO blood groups and multiple cancers. J. Amer. med. Ass. 185, 757 (1963).

HERVEY, G. W., L. K. DIAMOND, and VIRGINIA WATSON: Geographic blood group variability in the United States. J. Amer. med. Ass. 145, 80 (1951).

MAGATH, T. B., and J. BERKSON: Unpublished data.

TASWELL, H. F.: Unpublished data.

TSUKADA, Y., R. H. MOORE, I. D. J. BROSS, J. W. PICKREN, and E. COHEN: Blood groups in patients with multiple cancers. Cancer (Philad.) 17, 1229 (1964).

6. Leukemia or Lymphoma and Coexistent Primary Malignant Neoplasms

The case is, I think, clinically, an example of leukemia; but pathologically, of leukemia and cancer combined. April 2, 1878.

Thus did WHIPHAM conclude his observations on what was probably the first reported case of the coexistence of leukemia and another type of malignant lesion.

Almost 75 years later, the following case was encountered at the Mayo Clinic:

An Alaskan miner, 59 years old, was first seen at the clinic in 1947. He had no complaints and requested a general checkup. Examination revealed slightly enlarged axillary and cervical nodes. The leukocyte count was 37,000 per cubic millimeter of blood; 83 % were lymphocytes. The peripheral blood smear was characteristic of chronic lymphatic leukemia. A rotentgenogram of the thorax showed nothing abnormal. The patient was treated with roentgen rays over the cervical and axillary regions and the back. He returned at yearly intervals thereafter and remained asymptomatic until 1951.

At that time he stated he had lost 15 pounds (6.8 kg) in the past year but otherwise felt well. The leukocyte count was 255,000, 92 % of which were lymphocytes. Roentgenologic examination of the thorax revealed density in the medial portion of the right lung field just above the hilus (Fig. 3 A). This was interpreted by the roentgenologist and clinician as a widening of the mediastinum consistent with leukemia. The patient was given another course of roentgen therapy and dismissed.

Nine and one half months later, the patient returned complaining of cough, dyspnea, thoracic pain, weakness, anorexia, and continued loss of weight. The roentgenogram of the thorax at this time showed evidence of a poorly defined mass in the medial portion of the

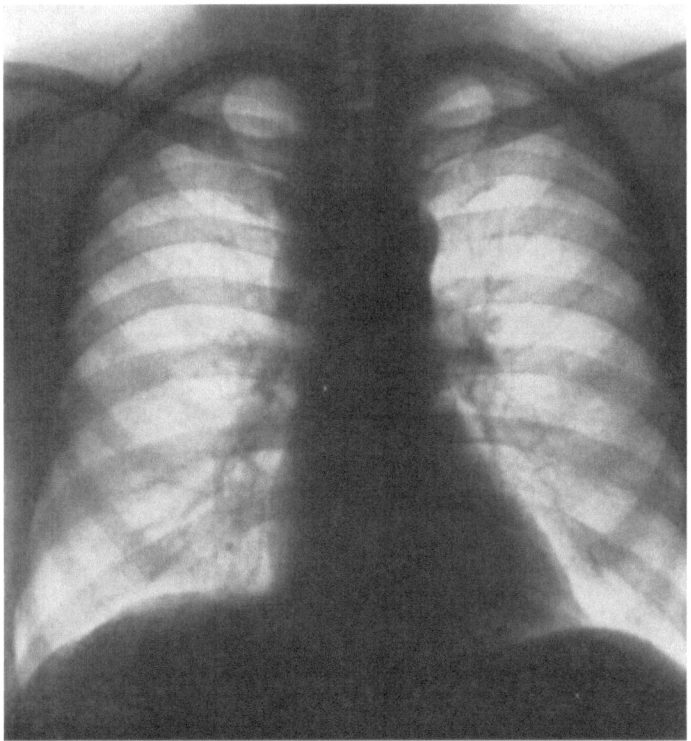

Fig. 3. *A*, Density in the medial portion of the right lung field interpreted as widening of the mediastinum secondary to leukemia

right lung with infiltration into the right upper lobe and right pleural effusion (Fig. 3 *B*). The patient was hospitalized and given more roentgen therapy, but his condition deteriorated with increased dyspnea and cyanosis and he died 1 month after admission. The clinician's impression at that time was that death was due to respiratory failure secondary to leukemic infiltration of the lungs.

Postmortem examination revealed scattered visceral infiltrations characteristic of lymphatic leukemia plus adenocarcinoma of high grade extensively involving the right lung and showing mediastinal and other more distal metastatic lesions.

This case, too, is "clinically, an example of leukemia; but pathologically, of leukemia and cancer combined."

Although the nature and location of the lesion in this case make it seem doubtful that even prompt surgical attack could have prolonged this patient's life, this is a striking example of the diagnostic enigma provided by the patient with diffuse reticuloendothelial malignant disease plus a second focally located malignant lesion. Superficially such a problem seems to be chiefly didactic — a perplexing challenge for the clinicopathologic conference. However, chronic leukemia or lymphoma may frequently run a benign course, and palliative measures may yield considerable benefit. It is not unusual for a patient with chronic leukemia or lymphoma to have 5 to 10 or more years of useful, productive life after the initial diagnosis is made. In such a patient, to interpret the signs and symptoms of a potentially curable

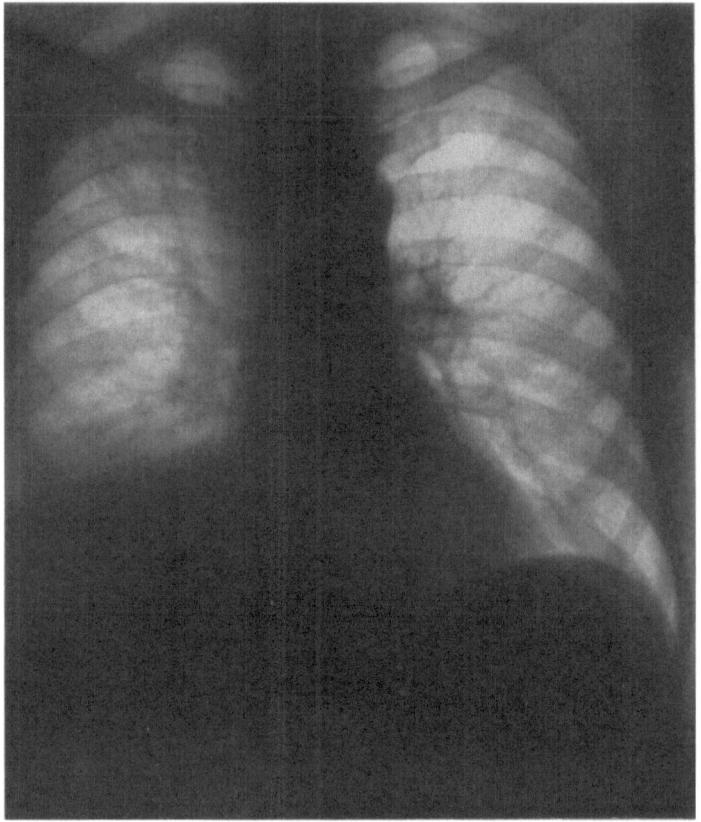

Fig. 3. *B*, Nine months later. Density in medial portion of the right lung field with infiltration in the right upper lobe and pleural effusion

independent, focal malignant lesion as a part of the generalized disease could have tragic consequences.

Much of the literature would lead the clinician to believe that a combination of leukemia or lymphoma plus a second focal malignant lesion is a freak occurrence that he may never see in a lifetime of practice. In 1944, MORRISON and associates report that in a series of 600 patients with leukemia they found only 2 (0.33 %) who had an additional malignant disease. They concluded that the coexistence of leukemia and other malignant disease is a "rare phenomenon." In later publications REISS and KONHEIM, and AXELROD and BERMAN have testified further to the rarity of the combination of these malignant conditions. In sharp contrast, however, is the more recent series reported by BERESFORD, in which 20 primary malignant lesions were found in 106 patients with leukemia, an incidence of 19 %. VIDEBAEK has stated, "the frequency of their coexistence is undoubtedly so high that it cannot be simply incidental." It is hoped that this presentation may in some measure resolve these apparent contradictions.

a) Cases Reported in the Literature

The cases classified and listed in Tables 11 and 12 were garnered from a careful review of the literature and seem to be valid examples of leukemia or lymphoma associated with another primary malignant lesion. It is of interest that over the past 2 decades there has been an almost exponential increase in the frequency with which such cases have been reported. In 1944 MORRISON and associates could find only 21 cases of primary malignant neoplasms occurring in association with leukemia in the world literature. Cases associated with lymphoma had been reported in

Table 11. *Review of the Literature: Leukemia Plus Malignant Neoplasms*

Type of malignant neoplasm	Cases	References
Chronic lymphatic leukemia	242	
Skin or lips	72	[6, 10, 14, 43, 50, 56, 59, 63, 69, 84, 88, 100, 102, 112, 126, 132, 143—145, 147, 166, 169, 170]
Colon and rectum	23	[10, 19, 56, 69, 78, 88, 107, 121, 123, 147, 169]
Stomach	22	[10, 13, 19, 20, 28, 36, 41, 49, 56, 88, 112, 118, 121, 125, 142, 156]
Lung	20	[10, 26, 54, 55, 62, 69, 80, 88, 89, 112, 119, 120, 144, 146, 160]
Cervix	13	[21, 36, 87, 88, 112, 151, 173, 174]
Prostate	12	[10, 23, 56, 68, 69, 78, 112, 121, 154]
Breast	11	[10, 42, 56, 69, 88, 111, 145—147]
Kaposi's sarcoma	11	[16, 32, 34, 37, 57, 76, 86, 136, 138, 141, 162]
Bladder	7	[10, 56, 100, 121, 147]
Larynx	7	[11, 18, 60, 100, 121, 156, 165]
Pancreas	5	[47, 56, 69, 107, 112]
Kidney	4	[56, 97, 100]
Malignant melanoma	4	[10, 50, 109, 169]
Uterus	4	[69, 87]
Tongue	3	[111, 146, 147]
Carcinoid	2	[120]
Esophagus	2	[5, 36]
Anus	1	[69]
Appendix	1	[112]
Hepatoma	1	[30]
Liver, bile ducts	1	[44]
Maxillary sinus	1	[108]
Multiple myeloma	1	[164]
Nose, adnexal carcinoma	1	[64]
Oral cavity	1	[56]
Parotid	1	[69]
Pleura, endothelioma	1	[53]
Sarcoma	1	[56]
Bladder plus skin	2	[71, 87]
Cervix plus lung	1	[93]
Fibrosarcoma plus prostate	1	[114]
Kidney plus lung	1	[98]
Leiomyosarcoma plus ovary	1	[169]
Neurofibrosarcoma plus skin	1	[92]
Colon plus lung plus prostate	1	[82]
Sarcoma plus skin plus vulva	1	[7]

Table 11 (Continued)

Type of malignant neoplasm	Cases	References
Chronic myelogenous leukemia	45	
Cervix	9	[50, 51, 174]
Skin	5	[56, 88, 167, 169]
Uterus	5	[56, 90, 174]
Lung	4	[36, 74, 119, 144]
Stomach	4	[24, 56, 74, 179]
Breast	3	[56, 169]
Brain, astrocytoma	2	[56, 144]
Colon and rectum	2	[8, 88]
Kaposi's sarcoma	2	[1, 158]
Jejunum	1	[8]
Hemangioendothelioma	1	[88]
Kidney	1	[74]
Liver	1	[54]
Ovary	1	[117]
Pancreas	1	[4]
Thyroid	1	[115]
Cervix plus kidney	1	[12]
Skin plus uterus	1	[155]
Acute leukemias	51	
Thyroid	11	[15, 40, 42, 79, 90, 122, 148]
Breast	10	[36, 56, 67, 98, 105, 134, 168]
Cervix	7	[151, 161, 169]
Colon or rectum	4	[36, 78, 98, 107]
Lung	3	[169]
Testis	3	[56, 105]
Ovary	2	[36, 56]
Skin	2	[36, 56]
Uterus	2	[56]
Bile ducts	1	[56]
Kidney, sarcoma	1	[75]
Malignant melanoma	1	[176]
Neuroastrocytoma	1	[131]
Ovary, teratocarcinoma	1	[29]
Stomach	1	[165]
Breast plus kidney	1	[93]
Leukemia, type unspecified	26	
Cervix	6	[82, 151]
Colon and rectum	5	[82, 123, 153]
Skin or lips	5	[96, 130]
Malignant melanoma	2	[82, 130]
Prostate	2	[82]
Breast	1	[130]
Larynx	1	[82]
Oral cavity	1	[82]
Pancreas	1	[171]
Pharynx	1	[82]
Retinoblastoma	1	[82]
Total	364	

Table 12. *Review of the Literature: Lymphoma Plus Malignant Neoplasms*

Type of malignant neoplasm	Cases	References
Lymphosarcoma	71	
Colon or rectum	20	[*35, 36, 78, 85, 98, 123, 124, 128, 129, 170*]
Skin or lips	11	[*45, 64, 94, 117, 126, 172*]
Kaposi's sarcoma	10	[*3, 9, 17, 73, 95, 99, 138, 152, 163*]
Lung	5	[*36, 98, 149, 170*]
Stomach	5	[*25, 43, 127, 140, 171*]
Prostate	3	[*36, 110*]
Ovary	2	[*45, 51*]
Vulva	2	[*43, 72*]
Anus	1	[*27*]
Breast	1	[*81*]
Esophagus	1	[*139*]
Larynx	1	[*67*]
Malignant melanoma	1	[*43*]
Penis	1	[*159*]
Thyroid	1	[*77*]
Breast plus uterus	1	[*39*]
Cervix plus skin	1	[*46*]
Colon plus kidney	1	[*150*]
Kidney plus stomach	1	[*61*]
Skin plus testis	1	[*51*]
Skin plus uterus	1	[*45*]
Hodgkin's disease	54	
Kaposi's sarcoma	22	[*3, 22, 37, 48, 51, 52, 66, 91, 99, 113, 130, 133, 157, 177, 178*]
Skin and lips	6	[*43, 130, 172*]
Colon and rectum	5	[*120, 130*]
Lung	3	[*58, 130, 135*]
Breast	2	[*130*]
Larynx	2	[*103, 130*]
Malignant melanoma	2	[*45, 130*]
Osteogenic sarcoma	2	[*130*]
Prostate	2	[*36, 130*]
Cervix	1	[*130*]
Ependymoma	1	[*130*]
Esophagus	1	[*130*]
Multiple myeloma	1	[*65*]
Pharynx	1	[*130*]
Thyroid	1	[*130*]
Uterus	1	[*130*]
Breast plus sarcoma	1	[*31*]
Reticulum cell sarcoma	15	
Colon and rectum	5	[*35, 36, 78*]
Breast	1	[*36*]
Kaposi's sarcoma	1	[*3*]
Kidney	1	[*108*]
Prostate	1	[*45*]
Skin	1	[*45*]
Tongue	1	[*36*]

Table 12 (Continued)

Type of malignant neoplasm	Cases	References
Vulva	1	[36]
Ileum, adenocarcinoma, 3 lesions	1	[33]
Esophagus plus liver	1	[2]
Lip plus skin	1	[14]
Follicular lymphoblastoma	3	
Kaposi's sarcoma	3	[99, 116]
Lymphoma, type unspecified	58	
Skin or lips	23	[96, 137]
Colon and rectum	6	[137]
Breast	4	[137]
Lung	4	[137]
Prostate	4	[137]
Cervix	3	[137]
Bladder	2	[96, 137]
Carcinoid	2	[137]
Kaposi's sarcoma	2	[116, 137]
Larynx	2	[137]
Stomach	1	[137]
Chondrosarcoma	1	[137]
Ependymoma	1	[137]
Kidney	1	[137]
Malignant melanoma	1	[137]
Tongue	1	[137]
Total	202	

approximately the same number. By 1957, we found that the combined total had risen to 194 cases (MOERTEL and HAGEDORN). Over the past 8 years this total has risen to 566, exclusive of the cases in this study.

The distribution of types of malignant neoplasms listed in Tables 11 and 12 show three exceptions to what might be expected in a random sampling of all patients with malignant neoplasms: (1) the remarkable frequency of coexistence of Kaposi's sarcoma, particulary with Hodgkin's disease, but also in the overall group of leukemias and lymphomas; (2) the preponderance of epitheliomas of the skin and lips in the chronic lymphatic leukemia group; and (3) the disproportionate representation of cancers of the thyroid and, to a lesser extent, cancers of the breast and cervix in the acute leukemia group. These points will be discussed later in this section.

b) Selection of Our Cases for Study

For study we selected cases of leukemia or lymphoma associated with another malignant lesion encountered at the Mayo Clinic in the 10 years from January 1, 1944, through December 31, 1953. All pathologic and hematologic findings were reviewed, and in any case in which the diagnosis was questionable the available material was reexamined. The presence of all lymphomas and other malignant lesions was proved at pathologic examination of specimens removed at operation or at autopsy; a clinical diagnosis alone was not sufficient evidence for inclusion of the case in the series. Cases in which the diagnosis was made elsewhere prior to examination at this clinic were included only if the pathologic diagnosis had been confirmed at the Mayo Clinic.

The diagnosis of leukemia was established in all cases included for study through examination of smears of peripheral blood or specimens of bone marrow or both. In any case in which the validity of the diagnosis could possibly be questioned on review of the hematologic reports, the hematologic specimens were reevaluated. The chief problem in this regard involved differentiation of leukemoid reactions from true leukemia. Myelocytic leukemoid reactions are not uncommon in the presence of malignant lesions, and in some cases the differentiation from myelogenous leukemia may be difficult or impossible. In a few of our cases the distinction could be made only by following the course of the patient or by the finding of leukemic infiltration at postmortem examination. All cases in which the diagnosis of leukemia could not be made with certainty were discarded from this series.

The diagnostic problem may rarely be complicated further by a lymphocytic leukemoid reaction due to malignant disease. The hematologic picture of leukemoid reaction in these cases is apparently indistinguishable from that in lymphatic leukemia. The diagnosis in the infrequently reported cases has been based on one of the following criteria: (1) the permanent reversion of the hematologic picture to normal after surgical removal of the malignant lesion, or (2) the absence of any evidence of leukemic infiltration at postmortem examination. This phenomenon was reviewed by KLEEMAN, who found five cases in the literature and reported one of his own. To our knowledge, this condition was not seen at our clinic during the period of this study.

In brief then, the 120 cases reported on herein are only those in which the coexistence of leukemia or lymphoma and other malignant disease seemed to be established beyond any reasonable doubt.

c) Leukemia Plus Malignant Lesions

Among the 2,134 patients with leukemia who were seen at the Mayo Clinic during the study period, there were 52 who had an additional primary malignant lesion. Thirty-six of these were men and 16 women. In 45 cases the associated malignant lesion was diagnosed surgically and in 7 at autopsy. In 27 cases the malignant lesion was diagnosed simultaneously with the diagnosis of leukemia, in 18 preceding the diagnosis of leukemia, and in 16 after the diagnosis of leukemia; in 1 case a primary malignant lesion was diagnosed simultaneously with the diagnosis of leukemia and another independent malignant lesion was diagnosed subsequently.

The average age at which leukemia was proved in the patients with the combined diseases was 63 years with a range from 30 to 79 years. The average age at which the existence of another malignant lesion was proved was 59 with a range from 30 to 79 years.

Data on these patients are presented in Table 13.

Table 13. *Type of Leukemia or Lymphoma and Type and Site of Associated Malignant Lesion in Our 120 Cases*

Malignant lesion and site	Leukemia: 52 cases				Lymphoma: 68 cases				Total
	Chronic Lymphatic	Myelogenous	Acute Lymphatic	Myelogenous	Follicular lymphoblastoma	Reticulum cell sarcoma	Hodgkin's disease	Lymphosarcoma	
Carcinoma									
Skin or lips (epithelioma)[1]	8[2]	3			1	3	1	11[3]	} 30
Skin and lips (epithelioma)					1		1		
Lip, adenocarcinoma								1	1
Mouth								1	1
Pharynx		1					1		2
Larynx	1								1
Parotid					1				1
Thyroid							1	1	2
Mandible	1								1
Breast	4	2					1	4[4]	11
Lung	2	1					1		4
Esophagus	1							1	2
Stomach	3			1		1	1	1	7
Colon or rectum	3		1	2				3	4	13
and skin		2						1	3
and rectum			1						1
and vulva								1	1
Kidney (hypernephroma)	2								2
Bladder	2	1						3	6
Prostate[5]	2	1	1		2	1	1	2	11
and skin	1								1
Penis								2	2
Ovary							1	1	2
Uterus	1						1	1	3
Cervix						1		2	3
Seminoma									
Testis				1					1
Testis and epitheliomas of skin and mouth								1	1
Teratoma, malignant, testis								1	1
Kaposi's sarcoma								1	1
and carcinoma of prostate								1	1
Melanoma, choroid					1				1
Skin								1	1
Neurilemmoma, cauda equina				1					1
Astrocytoma of brain							1		1
Total 2 [1,5]	31	11	3	5	6	7	13	42	120

[1] One case of acute stem cell leukemia.
[2] Single in 5; multiple in 3.
[3] Single in 8; multiple in 3.
[4] One bilateral.
[5] One case of acute monocytic leukemia.

d) Lymphoma Plus another Malignant Lesion

Among the 2,340 patients with malignant lymphoma seen at the Mayo Clinic from 1944 through 1953, there were 68 who an additional primary malignant lesion. Forty-three of these were male and 25 were female. In 61 cases the diagnosis of lymphoma was proved surgically and in 7 at autopsy. In 60 cases the additional malignant condition was diagnosed surgically and in 8 at autopsy. In 25 cases the malignant lesion was diagnosed simultaneously with the diagnosis of lymphoma, in 23 preceding the diagnosis of lymphoma, and in 17 after the diagnosis of lymphoma; 2 patients had preceding as well as simultaneous independent malignant lesions; and 1 patient had both preceding and subsequent independent malignant lesions.

The average age at time of diagnosis of lymphoma of the patients who had the combined diseases was 57 with a range of 12 to 82 years. The average age at diagnosis of the focal malignant condition was 57 with a range of 25 to 85 years.

Data on these patients are presented in Table 13.

Because it is of special interest, the following case is presented in more detail:

A white woman, 50 years old, was first seen at the Mayo Clinic on March 9, 1953, because of severe and persistent headache. Examination revealed bilateral papilledema and other neurologic signs suggesting an intracranial neoplasm. On March 12, a right frontoparietal craniotomy was performed with resection of a relatively well-localized astrocytoma of the right frontal lobe (Fig. 4 A). Following operation the patient was given intensive roentgen treatment to the right frontal, parietal, and temporal regions in several courses from March 20 to April 7.

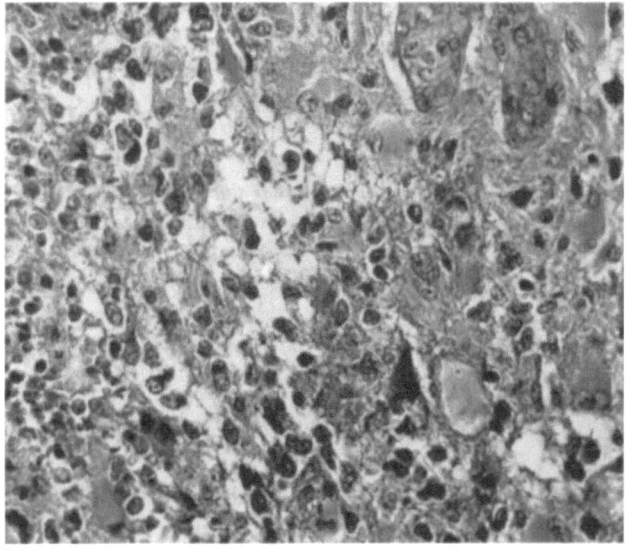

Fig. 4. A, Astrocytoma, grade 4 (glioblastoma multiforme), of the brain. (Hematoxylin and eosin; ×275.)

On July 17, 1953, the patient returned and stated she had felt well in the intervening 3 months. About 2 weeks before her return, however, she had noticed a small lump just above and in front of the right ear. Examination revealed a firm mass 3 cm in diameter just below the previous craniotomy scar and in the approximate center of one of the previous fields of roentgen therapy. One physician also recorded the presence of a firm, enlarged right cervical node. The mass was excised, and the pathologic diagnosis was reticulum cell sarcoma of the scalp, unquestionably different in morphology from the previous brain tumor (Fig. 4 B). The patient was given more roentgen therapy, but she died at home within the next 6 months. Autopsy was not performed.

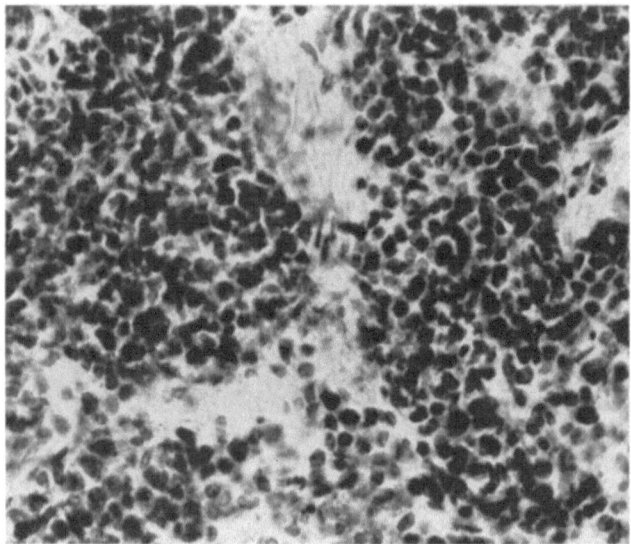

Fig. 4. B, Reticulum cell sarcoma removed from scalp of same patient 4 months after lesion was removed from the brain. (Hematoxylin and eosin; ×385.)

Certainly the possibility is strong that these two lesions occurred coincidentally and were entirely unrelated. However, the unusual combination of circumstances in this case tempts one to risk the post hoc ergo propter hoc fallacy and speculate as to the possible role that roentgen treatment may have played in the genesis of the subsequent reticulum cell sarcoma. If this speculation is true, it must indeed represent a rare occurrence, and to our knowledge no similar case has been reported in the literature.

From Table 13 it appears that the patients in this series show no significant difference in the distribution of types of malignancy from that which one would expect to find in a random sampling of the general population. No statistically valid evidence is presented in this series that leukemia or lymphoma predisposes to any other specific type of primary malignancy.

e) Coexistence of Kaposi's Sarcoma and Leukemia or Lymphoma

The prominent representation of Kaposi's sarcoma in Tables 11 and 12 is undoubtedly due in part to the special interest shown in this phenomenon by various reporting authors. It will be noted, however, that we have also presented two such cases (Fig. 5 and 6) in our consecutive series of 120 patients. These two cases represented only 1.67 % of the patients in our study with leukemia or lymphoma plus another primary malignant neoplasm; Kaposi's sarcoma, however, represented only 0.067 % of the 36,000 malignant neoplasms diagnosed at the Mayo Clinic during this same 10-year period. These same two cases represent an 8 % incidence of lymphoma among the 24 patients with Kaposi's sarcoma seen during this study period. The disproportionate coincidence of Kaposi's sarcoma and leukemia or lymphoma is not peculiar to this series alone. Of 41 patients with Kaposi's sarcoma

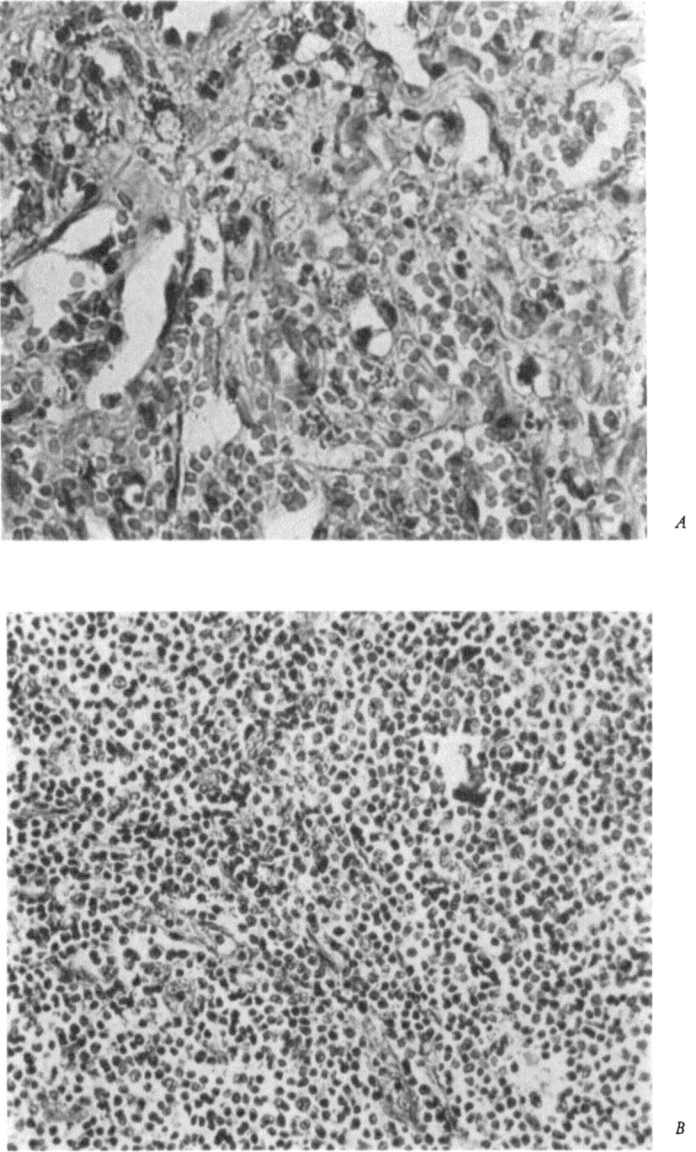

Fig. 5. *A*, Kaposi's sarcoma removed from skin of ankle. (Hematoxylin and eosin; ×400.) *B*, Lymphosarcoma in an axillary node. (Hematoxylin and eosin; ×350.)

reported by ALLEN, 7 (17 %) had associated lymphoma; and of 50 patients reported by Cox and HELWIG, 3 (6 %) had associated leukemia or lymphoma. In Africa, where both lymphoma and Kaposi's sarcoma are common, a similar association has been cited. Autopsy findings reported by LOTHE and MURRAY in 19 African patients with Kaposi's sarcoma revealed that 2 (11 %) had associated Hodgkin's disease. Of still greater significance are the cases reported by WILLIS, BELLONI, UYS and

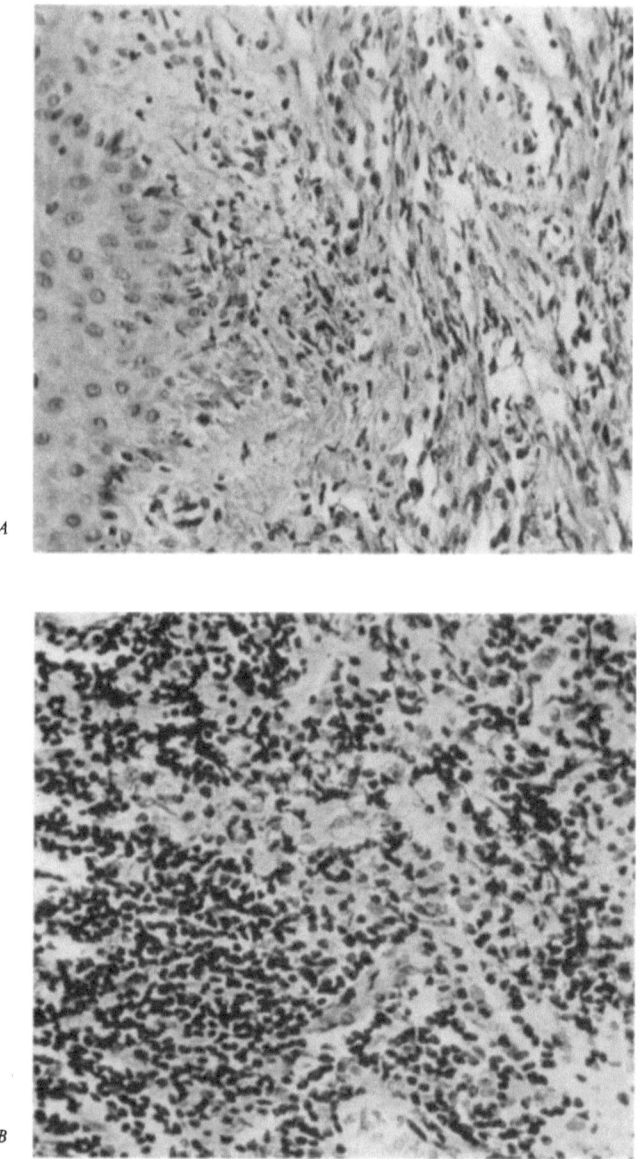

Fig. 6. *A*, Kaposi's sarcoma in skin of leg. (Hematoxylin and eosin; ×300.) *B*, Lymphosarcoma in a cervical node. (Hematoxylin and eosin; ×350.)

BENNETT, and LOTHE and MURRAY. In each of these there were various stages of transition between the typical histology of lymphoma and the typical histology of Kaposi's sarcoma in different specimens taken from the same patient.

Although there is some dispute, the largest body of the literature categorizes Kaposi's sarcoma as a neoplasm taking origin in the reticuloendothelial system. MONTGOMERY has pointed out the pathogenetic similarities between Kaposi's sarcoma and lymphoblastomatous involvement of the skin. He has stated that transitions between the two conditions might be expected.

It is well established that a patient with malignant lymphoma may present the microscopic picture of two or more specific types of lymphoma as well as various intermediate stages. The coexistence of lymphoma and leukemia in the same patient as so-called leukosarcoma is also not uncommon. It would seem reasonable, therefore, to assume that the picture of both Kaposi's sarcoma and leukemia or lymphoma in the same patient does not represent a true example of multiple primary malignant lesions but rather is a further extension of the pleomorphism of reticuloendothelial malignant disease.

The frequency of this phenomenon cannot be ignored; it provides strong evidence that Kaposi's sarcoma should be included in the leukemia-lymphoma spectrum of malignant diseases of the reticuloendothelial system.

f) Coexistence of Epitheliomas of the Skin and Chronic Lymphatic Leukemia

The most frequent malignant neoplasms occurring with chronic lymphatic leukemia, as reported in the literature as well as in this series, are epitheliomas of the skin and lips. These neoplasms are not found in such a predominance with other leukemias or with lymphomas. This observation has led to speculation in the literature that chronic lymphatic leukemia may predispose to the development of epithelial neoplasms of the skin or lips. The frequency with which chronic lymphatic leukemia and skin cancer are reported to coexist does not in itself, however, constitute satisfactory evidence of any predisposition to this occurrence. These patients are, in the main, elderly males, in whom a high rate of occurrence of skin cancer might be expected. Also, since patients with chronic lymphatic leukemia usually have relatively frequent medical observations over the long periods that the good prognosis of this disease usually allows, recognition and excision of small skin cancers would be more likely than in the general population or in patients with more fulminant types of malignant disease. To provide more substantial information on this relationship, GUNZ and ANGUS compared, in a retrospective study, the incidence of cancer of the skin among patients with chronic lymphatic leukemia seen at the Christchurch Hospital, Christchurch, New Zealand, with the expected incidence based on figures published by the New Zealand Cancer Registry. In the same way they also compared the incidence of chronic lymphatic leukemia among their skin cancer patients with the expected incidence. They concluded that the incidence of cancer of the skin showed a significant excess in patients with chronic lymphatic leukemia and also that skin cancer patients showed a statistically significant increase in the incidence of chronic lymphatic leukemia. A careful analysis of the methods used in this study, however, must raise a substantial doubt as to the validity of these conclusions. This was a retrospective study, and the pitfalls of such a study are manifest when one attempts to correlate the coincidence of two disease states. As has been pointed out earlier in this work, retrospective studies of this kind, when performed by different investigators, have sometimes led to diametrically opposed conclusions. The number of patients showing a coincidence of lymphatic leukemia and skin cancer in each part of their study was small — only 19 and 10, respectively. In several of their patients the diagnosis of skin cancer was made only on clinical observation without histologic confirmation. Even if this had been a prospective study in larger volume and all lesions had been confirmed pathologically, the nature of their control group would seem highly questionable. The rate of observation of skin cancers on patients of a single hospital population, made at least in part by investigators who have demonstrated for several years their interest in the coexistence of cancer and leukemia, can hardly be compared fairly with the rate at which all practicing physicians are likely to report these usually small and easily treatable lesions to a national tumor registry.

A methodology analogous to that of Gunz and Angus can be used to compare the relative frequency of major primary malignant neoplasms in leukemia patients as recorded in the Connecticut Cancer Case Registry with the overall distribution of primary malignant neoplasms recorded in the End Results Evaluation of the National Cancer Institute to which the Connecticut Registry is a major contributor. The results of such comparison are presented in Table 14. These figures would make it appear that in the United States carcinomas of the skin occurred in their expected proportion in leukemia patients whereas a predisposition exists to carcinoma of the prostate in males and to carcinoma of the large bowel and kidney in females. Such statistical maneuvering is, of course, completely invalid, and such conclusions are absurd.

Table 14. *Proportionate Distribution of Major Cancers in Leukemia Patients Compared With Overall Distribution of Cancer Registry Patients: An Example of Invalid Statistical Methodology*

Type of cancer	Male patients Cancer registry,[1] %	Leukemia patients,[2] %	Type of cancer	Female patients Cancer registry,[1] %	Leukemia patients,[2] %
Skin	22	25	Breast	33	12
Colon and rectum	22	12	Colon and rectum	19	37
Lung	19	12	Cervix	17	12
Prostate	15	33	Skin	12	12
Stomach	10	12	Ovary	6	12
Bladder	9	0	Stomach	5	0
Kidney	3	4	Bladder	3	0
			Lung	3	0
			Uterus	3	0
			Kidney	1	12

[1] Derived from End Results and Mortality Trends in Cancer (Cutler and Ederer).
[2] Derived from Mersheimer et al.

If a predisposition to epitheliomas of the skin exists in patients with chronic lymphatic leukemia, proof of such a predisposition must be obtained through a carefully controlled prospective study. No such work has, as yet, appeared in the literature.

g) Cancer and Acute Leukemias: Effects of Radiation

It may be noted in Table 11 that the malignant neoplasms most frequently reported in association with the acute leukemias are also those for which ionizing radiation is frequently used as a curative or palliative tool — carcinomas of the thyroid, breast, and cervix. The evidence suggesting that systemic ^{131}I therapy of metastatic thyroid carcinoma may have a causative effect in the induction of acute myelogenous leukemia has already been cited. The evidence concerning external radiation therapy, as is commonly used for carcinoma of the cervix or breast, is less conclusive. The frequency of reporting of these neoplasms with acute leukemia is due, at least in part, to the interest of medical authors in questioning the leukemogenic effect of therapeutic radiation therapy. No such case was observed at the Mayo Clinic during the 10-year period of our study, in spite of the fact that 3,818 patients with carcinoma of the breast or cervix were seen and that a large proportion of these received radiation therapy.

h) Incidence

The overall incidence of primary cancers occurring in patients with leukemia and lymphoma as reported in this series may only be considered as a minimal figure since it does not include patients who may have had a primary malignant lesion proved elsewhere either prior to, or subsequent to, their visits to the Mayo Clinic. Also, many of the patients have died without postmortem examination, and some are still alive. Probably a closer approximation of the true incidence is provided by a study of those patients with leukemia or lymphoma on whom postmortem examinations were performed. The incidence of independent primary malignant neoplasms in all cases of leukemia and lymphoma and the incidence in cases studied at autopsy are tabulated in Table 15. Included in the broad category of acute leukemia are all cases of acute lymphocytic, myelogenous, and monocytic leukemia as well as other more primitive-cell types of leukemia.

Table 15. *Incidence of Primary Malignant Neoplasms in Patients With Leukemia or Lymphoma Seen at the Mayo Clinic*

Type	All cases			Autopsy performed		
		Associated primary malignant lesion			Malignant lesion associated	
	Total	Cases	%	Total	Cases	%
Leukemia						
Acute	867	10	1.2	129	4	3.1
Chronic myelogenous	528	11	2.1	36	4	11.1
Chronic lymphatic	739	31	4.2	39	7	18.9
Total	2,134	52	2.4	204	17	8.3
Lymphoma						
Follicular lymphoblastoma	195	6	3.1	4	0	0
Reticulum cell sarcoma	368	7	1.9	40	2	5.0
Hodgkin's disease	826	13	1.6	92	5	5.4
Lymphosarcoma	951	42	4.4	65	6	9.2
Total	2,340	68	2.9	201	13	6.5
Grand total: Leukemia and lymphoma	4,474	120	2.7	405	30	7.4

The variation in incidence among the specific types of leukemia and lymphoma is most easily explained by the predominant age groups affected by these types, for example acute leukemia occurring more frequently in childhood and chronic lymphatic leukemia and lymphosarcoma occurring in the more cancer-prone (advanced or older) age group.

It is impossible to make a statistically valid comparison between the incidence of malignant disease in this series and that in the general population. This is because of the lack of an adequate control group and also because a large number of patients seen at the Mayo Clinic are referred and therefore any series reported is predetermined to be at least in part selected. In spite of these factors, however, the figures in Table 15 show beyond any doubt that the occurrence of an independent primary malignant lesion in a patient with leukemia or lymphoma is decidedly not a rarity. It probably equals and perhaps exceeds the occurrence among persons of comparable age in the general population.

i) Comment

The physician who deals with patients afflicted with leukemia or lymphoma must be constantly aware of the possibility of a coexistent malignant disease. This is especially true of the patients in whom the leukemia or lymphoma tends to run a relatively benign course. Any signs or symptoms suggestive of focal malignant lesion in a patient with leukemia or lymphoma should be regarded as representing a primary lesion until this has been proved otherwise pathologically.

Summary

A total of 566 cases of leukemia or lymphoma with coexistent primary malignant disease was found reported in the literature. To this we have added 120 cases from the files of the Mayo Clinic.

The following observations were made:

1. There is no statistically valid evidence that the presence of leukemia or lymphoma predisposes to the development of any other specific type of primary malignant neoplasm.

2. The incidence of another primary malignant lesion in patients with leukemia or lymphoma is probably comparable to, and perhaps exceeds, that in any segment of the general population of similar age.

3. The coexistence of Kaposi's sarcoma and leukemia or lymphoma in the same patient probably represents a morphologic variation of the same basic malignant disease of the reticuloendothelial system.

4. Any patient with leukemia or lymphoma who presents signs or symptoms of a focal malignant lesion should be regarded as having another primary lesion until this has been proved otherwise on pathologic examination.

References

[1] ABRAHAMSEN, A. M., and PER WETTELAND: Kaposis Sarkom og myelogen Leukemi. Nord. Med. 62, 1811 (1959).
[2] ALBRECHT, P.: Über die Multiplizität primärer maligner Geschwülste. Oncologia (Basel) 5, 12 (1952).
[3] ALLEN, A. C.: The Skin: A Clinicopathologic Treatise. St. Louis: C. V. Mosby Company 1954, p. 1000.
[4] ANGUS, H. B., and F. B. GUNZ: Chronic granulocytic leukemia and cancer. Blood 22, 88 (1963).

[5] ASKANAZY, M.: Leukämie und Tumoren. Schweiz. med. Wschr. 70, 29 (1940).

[6] AXELROD, A. R., and L. BERMAN: Multiple squamous cell carcinoma of the skin associated with chronic lymphatic leukemia: Observations on the effect of urethane therapy. Arch. Derm. Syph. (Chic.) 60, 625 (1949).

[7] BACH, W.: Tumorbereitschaft und Leukose. Zbl. Gynäk. 83, 1684 (1961).

[8] BARRET, W. D., K. T. MILLER, and C. R. FESSENMEYER: Multiple primary cancer: A study of thirty-six patients. Surg. Gynec. Obstet. 89, 767 (1949).

[9] BELLONI, L.: Maladie de Kaposi à évolution lymphosarcomateuse (contribution à l'étude des mésenchymopathies hyperplastico-néoplasiques). Ann. Derm. Syph. (Paris) 9, 45 (1949).

[10] BERESFORD, O. D.: Chronic lymphatic leukaemia associated with malignant disease. Brit. J. Cancer. 6, 339 (1952).

[11] BERK, M., and E. R. MOVITT: Leukemia complicated by cancer: Report of a case. Amer. J. clin. Path. 15, 246 (1945).

[12] BERNARD, JEAN, M. BOIRON, A. MANUS, C. JACQUILLAT, and J. RIPAULT: Épithélioma du col uterin, leucémie myéloïde chronique et épithélioma du rein chez la même malade. Presse méd. 72, 2675 1964).

[13] BICHEL, J.: Lymphatic leukemia and lymphatic leukemoid states in cancer of stomach. Blood 4, 759 (1949).

[14] BLACK, C. L., and S. CUMMINGS: Multiple malignancies of major importance occurring in the same individual. New Orleans med. surg. J. 103, 211 (1950).

[15] BLOM, P. S., A. QUERIDO, and C. H. W. LEEKSMA: Acute leukemia following x-ray and radioiodine treatment of thyroid carcinoma. Brit. J. Radiol. 28, 165 (1955).

[16] BLUEFARB, S. M.: Kaposi's Sarcoma: Multiple Idiopathic Hemorrhagic Sarcoma. Springfield, Ill.: Charles C. Thomas, Publisher 1957, p. 126.

[17] —, and J. R. WEBSTER: Kaposi's sarcoma associated with lymphosarcoma. Arch. intern. Med. 91, 97 (1953).

[18] BOURDIAL, J., Y. LALLEMANT, and W. SARFATI: Un cas de leucose survenue chez un malade opéré de laryngectomie totale. Ann. Oto-laryng. (Paris) 76, 983 (1959).

[19] BOUSSER, J., and G. MATHÉ: Association du cancer épithélial et de lymphomatose (leucosique ou non). Sem. Hôp. (Paris) 30, 821 (1954).

[20] BRENNER, A. J., and B. S. EPSTEIN: Lymphatic leukemia complicated by carcinoma of the stomach. Amer. J. Gastroent. 25, 116 (1956).

[21] BRÜCKNER: Lymphatische Leukämie und Portiocarcinom. Arch. Gynäk. 157, 616 (1934).

[22] BRUNNING, R. D., J. F. FOLEY, and I. E. FORTUNY: Hodgkin's disease and Kaposi's sarcoma: Report of a case. Arch. intern. Med. 112, 363 (1963).

[23] BUGHER, J. C.: Probability of chance occurrence of multiple malignant neoplasms. Amer. J. Cancer. 21, 809 (1934).

[24] BURG, K. M.: Ein mit Radiothor behandelter Fall von myeloischer Leukämie mit komplizierendem Magenkarzinom. Dtsch. med. Wschr. 1, 881 (1924).

[25] BURKE, M.: Multiple primary cancers. Amer. J. Cancer. 27, 316 (1936).

[26] CAHAN, W. G., F. S. BUTLER, W. L. WATSON, and J. L. POOL: Multiple cancers: Primary in the lung and other sites. J. thorac. Surg. 20, 335 (1954).

[27] CATTAN, R., and J. L. BONNETT: Cancer ano-rectal ictere hémolytique acquis: Stabilisation clinique apparition d'un diabète bronzé puis d'un lymphosarcome. Rev. méd.-chir. Mal. Foie 33, 157 (1958).

[28] —, and P. DELAVIERRE: Association d'un cancer gastrique et d'une leucémie lymphoïde, accompagnée d'anomalies des protéines sériques. Arch. Mal. Appar. dig. 47, 1226 (1958).

[29] CHALMERS, J. A.: Two cases of dysgerminoma ovarii, one occurring in a malignant teratoma in association with acute myelocytic leukaemia. J. Obstet. Gynaec. Brit. Emp. 57, 437 (1950).

[30] CLAY, A., G. CALVET, A. DEMAILLE, and L. ADENIS: Hépatome et leucose lymphoide. (Abstr.) Presse méd. 70, 2072 (1962).

[31] COHEN, HILLIARD, SIDNEY RUBIN, and GUSTAV EISEMANN: Hodgkin's disease (familial) associated with multiple malignant neoplasms. Cancer (Philad.) 11, 1247 (1958)

[32] COLE, H. N., and E. S. CRUMP: Report of two cases of idiopathic hemorrhagic sarcoma (Kaposi), the first complicated with lymphatic leukemia. Arch. Derm. Syph. (Chic.) 1, 283 (1920).

[33] COLLINS, J. J.: The occurrence of two or more primary malignant lesions. Radiology 32, 462 (1939).

[34] CONEJO-MIR: Quoted by Oettle, A. G.: Geographical and racial differences in the frequency of Kaposi's sarcoma as evidence of environmental or genetic causes. Acta Un. int. Cancr. 18, 330 (1962).

[35] CORNES, J. S.: Multiple primary malignant lymphomas and carcinomas of the intestinal tract in the same patient. J. clin. Path. 13, 483 (1960).

[36] —, T. G. JONES, and G. B. FISHER: The incidence of carcinoma in patients dying from leukaemia, malignant disorders of plasma cells, and malignant lymphoma. Brit. J. Cancer. 15, 200 (1961).

[37] COX, F. H., and E. B. HELWIG: Kaposi's sarcoma. Cancer (Philad.) 12, 289 (1959).

[38] CUTLER, S. J., and FRED EDERER: Part I. End results in cancer. In: End results and mortality trends in cancer. (National Cancer Institute Monograph 6.) U. S. Department of Health, Education, and Welfare, Public Health Service 1961, p. 5.

[39] DARLING, C. E.: Multiple primary malignancies with case illustrations. Grace Hosp. Bull. (Detroit) 26, 55 (1948).

[40] DARON, P., and P. PIZZOLATO: Acute myelogenous leukemia with giant cell carcinoma of thyroid. Arch. Path. 51, 72 (1951).

[41] DEENSTRA, H., M. C. VERLOOP, and A. DE MINJER: Lymphatische Leucaemie en Kanker. Ned. T. Geneesk. 93, 326 (1949).

[42] DELARUE, J., M. TUBIANA, and J. DUTREIX: Cancer de la thyroïde traité par l'iode radioactif: Terminaison par une leucédie aiguë après une amélioration importante. Bull. Ass. franç. Cancer 40, 263 (1953).

[43] DELCOURT, R.: Les tumeurs doubles à tissus histologiquement différents. Bull. Ass. franç. Cancer 31, 128 (1943).

[44] —, and P. VAN VLEIT: Coexistence d'une leucémie lymphoïde et d'un carcinom. Acta med. scand. 119, 47 (1944).

[45] DESAIVE, P.: Considérations statistiques et anatomo-cliniques à propos de 207 cas de cancers multiples. Rev. belge Path. 18, 173 (1947).

[46] —, J. FIRKET, M. CHEVREMONT, and A. DARDENNE: Contribution à l'étude des cancers multiples non systématisés. Bull. Ass. franç. Cancer 28, 6 (1939).

[47] DEWAN, C. H., and A. L. HUNTER, JR.: Multiple primary malignant tumors: A review with a case report. Guthrie Clin. Bull. (Sayre) 16, 71 (1946).

[48] DONELLY, W. J. (Ed.): Clinicopathologic conference: Hodgkin's disease and mucocutaneous lesions. Postgrad. Med. 33, 301 (1963).

[49] DUSTIN, P., JR.: Coexistence d'une leucémie lymphoïde et d'un carcinome gastrique. Rev. belge Sci. méd. 13, 199 (1941).

[50] ENGELBRETH-HOLM, J.: Leukaemi og anden malign svulst hos samme patient. Nord. Med. 9, 791 (1941).

[51] EPSTEIN, ERVIN: Extracutaneous manifestations of Kaposi's sarcoma: A systemic lymphoblastoma. Calif. Med. 87, 98 (1957).

[52] ERF, L.: Quoted by Greenstein, R. H., and A. S. Conston: Co-existent Hodgkin's disease and Kaposi's sarcoma: Report of a case with unusual clinical features. Amer. J. med. Sci. 218, 384 (1949).

[53] EVANS, T. S., M. Y. SWIRSKY, and H. M. CHERNOFF: Primary endothelioma of pleura: Report of case in patient with chronic lymphatic leukemia. Ann. intern. Med. 24, 262 (1946).

[54] —, L. WATERS, B. HARDIN, W. MATOSSIAN, E. GOLTRA, and V. DE LUCA: Carcinome primitif du foie, apparu chez un sujet atteint de leucémie myéloïde traitée par l'uréthane. Rev. Hémat. 6, 148 (1951).

[55] EVEN, R., J. VIBERT, and M. OURY: Leucémie lymphoïde et cancer du poumon. Paris méd. 139, 141 (1950).

[56] FABER, M., and K. BORUM: Leukaemia and a malignant tumour in the same patient. Brit. J. Haemat. 8, 313 (1962).

[57] FISCHER, J. W., and D. M. COHEN: Simultaneous occurrence of Kaposi's sarcoma, leukemia, and diabetes mellitus: Report of a case. Amer. J. clin. Path. 21, 586 (1951).

[58] FISCHER, W.: Kombination von Lymphogranulomatose, Tuberkulose und malignem Tumor in Lunge und Lymphknoten. Zbl. allg. Path. path. Anat. 86, 257 (1950).

[59] FUHS: Multizentrische Basalzellenepitheliome bei lymphatischer Leukämie. Derm. Wschr. 85, 1553 (1927).

[60] FUSI, G.: Considerazioni su di una rara associazione morbosa in un caso di reticolo-sarcoma ghiandolare irradiato; evoluzione emopatica del processo e coesistenza de un epithelioma laringeo. Radiol. med. (Torino) 41, 594 (1955).

[61] GALLAGHER, N. G., and R. H. MICKS: Multiple primary malignant disease with meningeal carcinomatosis. J. Irish med. Ass. 51, 115 (1962).

[62] GENÉVRIER, LORRAIN, and COIRRE: Lymphadénome leucémique associé à un épithélioma du poumon. Arch. méd.-chir. Appar. resp. 5, 195 (1930).

[63] GERTLER: Lymphatische Leukämie bei gleichzeitigen Haut-Carcinomen. Zbl. Haut-u. Geschl.-Kr. 68, 271 (1942).

[64] GRAHAM, J. H., and E. B. HELWIG: Bowen's disease and its relationship to systemic cancer. Arch. Derm. (Chic.) Syph. 80, 133 (1959).

[65] GREENBERG, B. B., D. STATS, and M. GOLDBERG: Simultaneous occurrence of plasma cell multiple myeloma and Hodgkin's disease. N. Y. med. 50, 305 (1950).

[66] GREENSTEIN, R. H., and A. S. CONSTON: Co-existent Hodgkin's disease and Kaposi's sarcoma: Report of a case with unusual clinical features. Amer. J. med. Sci. 218, (1949).

[67] GRIVOT, M., L. LEROUX, and R. CAUSSÉ: Présentation d'un malade chez lequel évoluent simultanément un épithélioma épidermoïde d'une corde vocale et un lympho-sarcome de la base de la lange. Presse méd. 1, 437 (1926).

[68] GUICHARD, A., R. ALEX, J.-L. VAUZELLE, R. LOIRE, and J.-F. DIDIERLAURENT: L'asso-ciation épithélioma leucemie leuco-carcinomes et carcino-leucémies. Lyon méd. 210, 395 (1963).

[69] GUNZ, F. W.: Leukaemia in New Zealand and Australia. Path. et Microbiol. (Basel) 27, 697 (1964).

[70] —, and H. B. ANGUS: Leukemia and cancer in the same patient. Cancer (Philad.) 18, 145 (1965).

[71] HALPERT, BELA, R. P. FOSTER, and M. J. MUSSER: Multiple malignant neoplasms in a man aged 89 years: A clinicopathologic conference. Geriatrics 14, 194 (1959).

[72] HARBITZ, F.: Über das gleichzeitige Auftreten mehrerer selbständig wachsender ("mul-tipler") Geschwülste. Beitr. path. Anat. 62, 503 (1916).

[73] HIGGINS, G. K.: Skin: Kaposi tumor. Brooklyn Hosp. J. 9, 187 (1951).

[74] HILGERT, H.: Über das Zusammentreffen von malignem Neubildungen untereinander und mit Krankheiten nicht sekundärer Art, nebst einigen weiteren statistischen Bei-trägen zur Krebsfrage. Z. Krebsforsch. 49, 390 (1939).

[75] HOTZ, A.: Zur Differentialdiagnose: Agranulocytose — Leukämie. Z. Kinderheilk. 62, 529 (1941).

[76] HUFNAGEL, L., and A. DUPONT: Sarcomatose idiopathique de Kaposi et leucémie lymphoïde. Bull. Soc. franç. Derm. Syph. 38, 656 (1931).

[77] HURT, H. H., and A. C. BRODERS: Multiple primary malignant neoplasms. J. Lab. clin. Med. 18, 765 (1933).

[78] HYMAN, G. A., J. E. ULTMANN, and C. A. SLANETZ: Chronic lymphocytic leukemia or lymphoma and carcinoma of the colon: Correlation with blood type A. J. Amer. med. Ass. 186, 1053 (1963).

[79] JELLIFFE, A. M., and K. M. JONES: Leukaemia after I[131] therapy for thyroid cancer. Clin. Radiol. 11, 134 (1960).

[80] JOSELEVICH, MIGUEL, LEON SUCARI, and MARCOS KLEIMANS: La asociacon del cancer y la leucemia. Pren. méd. argent. 45, 2154 (1958).

[81] JUDSON, H. A.: Simultaneous lymphosarcomatosis and carcinoma of the breast in the same individual: Case report. Radiology 29, 578 (1937).

[82] KLATTE, E. C., JACK YARDLEY, E. B. SMITH, ROBERT ROHN, and J. A. CAMPBELL: The pulmonary manifestations and complications of leukemia. Amer. J. Roentgen. **89**, 598 (1963).

[83] KLEEMAN, C. R.: Lymphocytic leukemoid reaction associated with primary carcinoma of breast. Amer. J. Med. **10**, 522 (1951).

[84] KREBS, A., and K. SCHWARZ: Besonders bösartiger, metastasierender Verlauf von Hautkarzinomen bei chronisch-lymphatischer Leukämie. Schweiz. med. Wschr. **93**, 15 (1963).

[85] KREIBIG, W.: Über multiple Geschwulstbildung im Darmtrakt. Dtsch. Z. Chir. **219**, 334 (1929).

[86] LANE, C. G., and A. M. GREENWOOD: Lymphoblastoma (mycosis fungioides) and hemorrhagic sarcoma of Kaposi in the same person. Arch. Derm. Syph. (Chic.) **27**, 643 (1933).

[87] LANNOIS, M., and C. REGAUD: Coexistence de la leucocythémie vraie et d'un cancer épithélial. Arch. Méd. exp. **7**, 254 (1895).

[88] LAWRENCE, J. H., and W. G. DONALD, JR.: The incidence of cancer in chronic leukemia and in polycythemia vera. Amer. J. med. Sci. **237**, 488 (1959).

[89] LECHELLE, P., S. VIALARD, and ROSEY: Un cas de leucémie lymphoïde chronique sans splénomégalie ni adénopathie périphérique, évoluant de pair avec un cancer suppuré du poumon. Bull. Soc. méd. Hôp. (Paris) **62**, 168 (1946).

[90] LEWALLEN, C. G., and J. T. GODWIN: Acute myelogenous leukemia complicating radioactive iodine therapy of thyroid cancer: Report of a case. Amer. J. Roentgen. **89**, 610 (1963).

[91] LOTHE, F., and J. F. MURRAY: Kaposi's sarcoma: Autopsy findings in the African. Acta Un. int. Cancr. **18**, 429 (1962).

[92] MACDONALD, ELEANOR J.: Occurrence of multiple primary cancers in a population of 200,000. Acta Un. int. Cancr. **16**, 1702 (1960).

[93] MÄHR, G., and R. P. KÖNIGSTEIN: Leukämie und zweifach primäre Neoplasie. Wien. Z. inn. Med. **43**, 353 (1962).

[94] MAJOR, R. H.: Multiple primary malignant tumors: With report of a case of carcinoma and sarcoma in the same individual. Bull. Johns Hopk. Hosp. **29**, 223 (1918).

[95] MALKINSON, F. D., and BERNARD STONE: Kaposi sarcomas, lymphoblastoma and herpes zoster. (Abstr.) Arch. Derm. Syph. (Chic.) **72**, 79 (1955).

[96] MALMIO, KAI: Multiple primary cancer: A clinical-statistical investigation based on 650 cases. Ann. Chir. Gynaec. Fenn. **48** (suppl. 92), 1 (1959).

[97] MARISCHLER, J.: Ein Fall von lymphatischer Leukämie und einem Grawitz'schen Tumor der rechten Niere. Wien. klin. Wschr. **9**, 686 (1896).

[98] MAUTNER, L. S.: Synchronous lymphatic leukaemia, bronchogenic carcinoma and hypernephroma. Canad. med. Ass. J. **63**, 66 (1950).

[99] McCARTHY, W. D., and G. T. PACK: Malignant blood vessel tumors: A report of 56 cases of angiosarcoma and Kaposi's sarcoma. Surg. Gynec. Obstet. **91**, 465 (1950).

[100] McMANUS, R. G., and S. C. SOMMERS: Significance of gastric polyps accompanying cancer. Amer. J. clin. Path. **23**, 746 (1953).

[101] MERSHEIMER, W. L., ABRAHAM RINGEL, and HENRY EISENBERG: Some characteristics of multiple primary cancers. Ann. N. Y. Acad. Sci. **114**, 896 (1964).

[102] MEYER-LAACK, H.: Leukamie und Karzinomgenese. Arch. Geschwulstforsch. **3**, 18 (1951).

[103] MILLS, W. H., R. DOMINGUEZ, and J. W. McCALL: Simultaneous carcinoma and malignant lymphoma of the larynx: Case report and review of literature. Laryngoscope (St Louis) **57**, 491 (1947).

[104] MOERTEL, C. G., and A. B. HAGEDORN: Leukemia or lymphoma and coexistent primary malignant lesions: A review of the literature and a study of 120 cases. Blood **12**, 788 (1957).

[105] MOLONEY, W. C.: Leukemia and exposure to x-ray: A report of 6 cases. Blood **14**, 1137 (1959).

[106] MONTGOMERY, H.: Mycosis fungoides, lymphoblastoma of the skin and allied conditions as general diseases. In Christian, H. A.: Oxford Medicine. New York: Oxford Univ. Press 1950, vol. 4, pt. 1. pp. 44(1)—44(20—23).

[107] MORRISON, M., F. FELDMAN, and A. A. SAMWICK: Carcinoma and leukemia: Report of two cases with combined lesions; review of literature. Ann. intern. Med. 20, 75 (1944).

[108] MOUNIER-KUHN, P., J. GAILLARD, J.-P. REBATTU, and B. JAKUBOWICZ: Statistique des cancers multiples à la clinique oto-rhino-laryngologique de Lyon de 1950 à 1962. Lyon méd. 212, 1389 (1964).

[109] NADBATH, R. P., and H. G. BULLWINKEL: Coexistence of intraocular melanoma and lymphatic leukemia. Arch. Ophthal. 48, 349 (1952).

[110] OPHÜLS, W.: A Statistical Survey of Three Thousand Autopsies. Stanford University: Stanford Univ. Press 1926, p. 316.

[111] ORTEGA, P., JR., I. Y. LI, and M. SHIMKIN: Metastasis of neoplasms to other neoplasms. Ann. West. Med. & Surg. 5, 601 (1951).

[112] OSBORNE, E. D., J. W. JORDON, F. C. HOAK, and F. J. PSCHIERER: Nitrogen mustard therapy in cutaneous blastomatous disease. J. Amer. med. Ass. 135, 1123 (1947).

[113] OSGOOD, E. E., and A. J. SEAMAN: Treatment of chronic leukemias. J. Amer. med. Ass. 150, 1372 (1952).

[114] OVNBØL, ANKER, and KNUD TERKILDSEN: Et tilfaelde af sarcom, carcinom og leukose hos samme patient. Nord. Med. 20, 1662 (1943).

[115] OZARDA, A., U. ERGIN, and M. A. BENDER: Chronic myelogenous leukemia following I-131 therapy for metastatic thyroid carcinoma: Report of a case and some considerations on etiologic factors. Amer. J. Roentgen. 85, 914 (1961).

[116] PACK, G. T., and J. DAVIS: Concomitant occurrence of Kapcsi's sarcoma and lymphoblastoma. Arch. Derm. Syph. (Chic.) 69, 604 (1954).

[117] PELLER, S.: Metachronous multiple malignancies in 5,876 cancer patients. Amer. J. Hyg. 34, 1 (1941).

[118] PENZOLD, H.: Leukämie und Carcinom. Dtsch. Arch. klin. Med. 180, 430 (1937).

[119] PETRAKIS, N. L., H. R. BIERMAN, K. H. KELLY, L. P. WHITE, and M. B. SHIMKIN: Effect of 1,4-dimethanesulfonyloxybutane (GT-41 or myleran) upon leukemia. Cancer (Philad.) 7, 383 (1954).

[120] PETRI, S.: Quoted by Bichel, J. [13].

[121] PISCIOTTA, A. V., and J. S. HIRSCHBOECK: Therapeutic considerations in chronic lymphocytic leukemia: Special reference to the natural course of the disease. Arch. intern. Med. 99, 334 (1957).

[122] POCHIN, E. E.: The occurrence of leukaemia following radioiodine therapy. In PITT-RIVERS, ROSALIND: Advances in thyroid research: Transactions of the Fourth International Goitre Conference, London, July, 1960. New York: Symposium Publications Division, Pergamon Press 1961, pp. 392—397.

[123] POLK, H. C., JR., J. S. SPRATT, JR., and H. R. BUTCHER, JR.: Frequency of multiple primary malignant neoplasms associated with colorectal carcinoma. Amer. J. Surg. 109, 71 (1965).

[124] POSTLETHWAIT, R. W., J. E. ADAMSON, and DERYL HART: Carcinoma of the colon and rectum. Surg. Gynec. Obstet. 106, 257 (1958).

[125] POTOCZEK, STANISLAW, LUDMILA HIRNLOWA, ALEKSANDER GIERMAŃSKI, and KAROL KAWECKI: Współistnienie przewlikłej białaczki limfatycznej i raka źoladka. Pol. Tyg. lek. 16 (pt. 2), 1408 (1961).

[126] PULVERTAFT, R. J. V.: Multiple primary epithelioma in lymphatic leukaemia. Brit. J. Surg. 24, 50 (1936).

[127] RABINOVITCH, J., B. PINES, and D. GRAYZEL: Coexisting lymphosarcoma and ulcer-carcinoma of the stomach. Arch. Surg. 64, 185 (1952).

[128] RABSON, S. M., P. L. STIER, J. C. BAUMGARTNER, and D. ROSENBAUM: Metastasis of cancer to cancer. Amer. J. clin. Path. 24, 572 (1954).

[129] RANKIN, T. J.: Multiple malignancies: Carcinoma of the colon and multicentric lymphosarcoma with recovery. J. Kans. med. Soc. 63, 99 (1962).

[130] RAZIS, D. V., H. D. DIAMOND, and L. F. CRAVER: Hodgkin's disease associated with other malignant tumors and certain non-neoplastic diseases. Amer. J. med. Sci. **238**, 327 (1959).

[131] REGELSON, WILLIAM, I. D. J. BROSS, JULIET HANANIAN, and GORYUN NIGOGOSYAN: Incidence of second primary tumors in children with cancer and leukemia: A seven-year survey of 150 consecutive autopsied cases. Cancer (Philad.) **18**, 58 (1965).

[132] REISS, F., and W. KONHEIM: Basal squamous cell epithelioma associated with leukemia. Arch. Derm. Syph. (Chic.) **55**, 507 (1947).

[133] REYNOLDS, W. A., R. K. WINKELMANN, and E. H. SOULE: Kaposi's sarcoma: A clinico-pathologic study with particular reference to its relationship to the reticuloendothelial system. Medicine (Baltimore) **44**, 419 (1965).

[134] ROATH, S., M. C. ISRAËLS, and J. F. WILKINSON: The acute leukemias: A study of 580 patients. Quart. J. Med. **33**, 256 (1964).

[135] RONCALLO, E., and G. PELUFFO: Su di un caso di associazione di carcinoma polmonare primitivo con metastasi ghiandolari e granuloma maligno addominale. Pathologica. **39**, 231 (1947).

[136] ROSEN, I.: Idiopathic hemorrhagic sarcoma and lymphatic leukemia. Arch. Derm. Syph. (Chic.) **48**, 566 (1943).

[137] ROSENBERG, S. A., H. D. DIAMOND, B. JASLOWITZ, and L. F. CRAVER: Lymphosarcoma: A review of 1269 cases. Medicine (Baltimore) **40**, 31 (1961).

[138] ROTHMAN, S.: Some clinical aspects of Kaposi's sarcoma in the European and North American population. Acta Un. int. Cancr. **18**, 364 (1962).

[139] ROUBIER, C.: Quelques observations de cancers primitifs multiples chez le même individu. Lyon méd. **189**, 69 (1953).

[140] SAAR: Quoted by Kreibig, W. [85].

[141] SACHS, W., and M. GRAY: Kaposi's sarcoma and lymphatic leukemia: Report of a case with histologic evidence of the two diseases in the same lesion. Arch. Derm. Syph. (Chic.) **51**, 325 (1945).

[142] SAUPE, E.: Bestrahlungswirkung bei gleichzeitiger Erkrankung an aleukämischer Lymphadenose und metastasierendem Magenkarzinom. Wien. klin. Wschr. **49**, 1104 (1936).

[143] SCHEUFFLER, A.: Carcinobildung auf einem Leukämid. Arch. Derm. Syph. (Berlin) **168**, 586 (1933).

[144] SCHILLING, R. F., and O. O. MEYER: Treatment of chronic granulocytic leukemia with 1,4-dimethanesulfonyloxybutane (myleran). New. Engl. J. Med. **254**, 986 (1956).

[145] SCHREINER, B. F., and W. H. WEHR: Cancer associated with leukemia. Amer. J. Cancer. **21**, 368 (1934).

[146] SCOTT, R. B.: The place of radiotherapy in the treatment of chronic lymphoid leukaemia. J. Fac. Radiol. (Lond.) **1**, 61 (1949).

[147] — Leukaemia. Lancet **1**, 1162 (1957).

[148] SEIDLIN, S. M., EDWARD SIEGEL, A. A. YALOW, and S. MELAMED: Acute myeloid leukemia following prolonged iodine-131 therapy for metastatic thyroid carcinoma. Science **123**, 800 (1956).

[149] SFORZA, M., and M. PERELLI-ERCOLINI: Du casi di tumori maligni doppi. Osped. maggiore **58**, 899 (1963).

[150] SHAPIRO, A. L., and H. BOLKER: Triple primary malignancy. Amer. J. Cancer. **40**, 441 (1940).

[151] SIMON, NORMAN, MARSHALL BRUCER, and RAYMOND HAYES: Radiation and leukemia in carcinoma of the cervix. Radiology **74**, 905 (1960).

[152] SIMPSON, C. LENORE, WILLIAM REGELSON, and FRANZ LESSMAN: Clinicopathologic conference. N. Y. St. J. Med. **59**, 4589 (1959).

[153] SLAUGHTER, D. P.: The multiplicity of origin of malignant tumors. Int. Abstr. Surg. **79**, 89 (1944).

[154] STANLEY, D. A.: Leukaemia and oestrogen therapy. Brit. med. J. **1**, 1460 (1957).

[155] STICH, W., and H. LANGHAMMER: Multiple Karzinome und Leukämie: Gemeinsames Vorkommen von Hautkarzinom, Uteruskarzinom und chronischer myeloischer Leukämie. Münch. med. Wschr. **103**, 502 (1961).

[156] SVEJDA, J.: Quoted by Bichel, J. [13].

[157] TALBOTT, J. H.: Clinical manifestations of Hodgkin's disease. N. Y. St. J. Med. 47, 1883 (1947).

[158] TEDESCHI, C. G., H. F. FOLSOM, and T. J. CARNICELLI: Visceral Kaposi's disease. Arch. Path. 43, 335 (1947).

[159] THALMESSINGER, V.: Quoted by Major, R. H. [94].

[160] THEMEL, K. G.: Über das Zusammentreffen von Bronchialkarzinom und Leukämie. Medizinische 1, 186 (1955).

[161] THIERY, M., and S. RINGOIR: Leucemie als mogelijke verwikkeling van Stralenbehandeling van Portiocarcinoom. Belg. T. Geneesk. 17, 524 (1961).

[162] THIJS, A.: Quoted by Oettle, A. G.: Geographical and racial differences in the frequency of Kaposi's sarcoma as evidence of environmental or genetic causes. Acta Un. int. Cancr. 18, 330 (1962).

[163] UYS, C. J., and M. B. BENNETT: Kaposi's sarcoma: A neoplasm of reticular origin. S. Afr. J. Lab. clin. Med. 5, 39 (1959).

[164] VANDER, J. B., and H. A. JOHNSON: Chronic lymphatic leukemia and multiple myeloma in the same patient. Ann. intern. Med. 53, 1052 (1960).

[165] VARSHAVSKII, A. G.: Association of leukemia with cancer (3 observations). Vop. Onkol. 8, 87 (1962).

[166] VIDEBAEK, A.: Heredity in human leukemia and its relation to cancer: A genetic and clinical study of 209 probands. Copenhagen: Arnold Busck 1947, pp. 83—85.

[167] VILČEK, E.: Koincidencia leukémie S. primárnou multiplicitou rakoviny Kože. Čs. Rentgenol. 18, 54 (1964).

[168] VOLL, ARTUR, and JOHANNES TVEIT: Levkemi hos tidligere Røntgen radium-behandlete Pasienter. Nord. Med. 58, 1114 (1957).

[169] WARREN, S., and T. EHRENREICH: Multiple primary malignant tumors and susceptibility to cancer. Cancer Res. 4, 554 (1944).

[170] —, and O. GATES: Multiple primary malignant tumors: A survey of the literature and a statistical study. Amer. J. Cancer. 16, 1358 (1932).

[171] WARWICK, T.: Discussion. Proc. roy. Soc. Med. 24, 206 (1930).

[172] WATSON, T. A.: Incidence of multiple cancer. Cancer (Philad.) 6, 365 (1953).

[173] WEINER, J. J., and A. M. SALA: Chronic lymphatic leukemia: Associated with carcinoma. J. Abdom. Surg. 3, 15 (1961).

[174] WENIG, H., and H. LANGE: Leukämie und Genitalkarzinom. Zbl. Gynäk. 80, 925 (1958).

[175] WHIPHAM, T.: Splenic leukaemia with carcinoma. Trans. path. Soc. Lond. 29, 313 (1878).

[176] WIESINGER, HERBERT, G. W. PHIPPS, and DU PONT GUERRY, III: Bilateral melanoma of the choroid associated with leukemia and meningioma. Arch. Ophthal. 62, 889 (1959).

[177] WILLIS, R. A.: Pathology of tumours. St. Louis: C. V. Mosby Company 1948, p. 780.

[178] WOLF, JACK: Discussion (idiopathic hemorrhagic sarcoma and lymphatic leukemia). Arch. Derm. Syph. (Chic.) 48, 566 (1943).

[179] ZADEK, I.: Radiothorium bei leukämischer Myelose: Grosse Dosierungen. Folia haemat. (Lpz.) 49, 287 (1933).

7. Carcinoid Tumors of the Small Intestine and Second Primary Cancers

During the course of this study, it was noted that an unusually high percentage (16 of 61, or 26%) of patients with carcinoid tumors of the small intestine were found to have second primary cancers of different tissues of origin. The total number of carcinoid patients was relatively small, and we could not rule out the chance occurrence of this high proportion of second cancers. To further pursue this matter, we studied all patients with carcinoid tumors of the small intestine seen at the Mayo Clinic before January 1, 1958 (MOERTEL and associates). It will be seen in Table 16 that the rate of occurrence of second cancers in the surgical group was 17% and in the autopsy group, 36%. These figures are quite striking when they are compared with the overall occurrence rates of multiple cancers of different tissues of origin observed in this study (2.3% and 8.1%, respectively). The specific types of cancer

Table 16. *Second Primary Malignant Neoplasms in Patients with Carcinoid Tumors of the Small Intestine*

Source of patients	Total patients	Patients with second cancer Number	%
Surgery	72	12	17
Autopsy	137	49	36
Total	209	61	29

found in these patients are listed in Table 17. The high rate of occurrence of second primary malignant neoplasms in patients with small-intestinal carcinoid tumors is

Table 17. *Site and Structure of Associated Primary Malignant Neoplasms in 61 of 209 Patients With Carcinoid Tumors of the Small Intestine*

Second Primary Lesion	Cases
Colon or rectum, adenocarcinoma	12
Stomach, adenocarcinoma	9
Breast, adenocarcinoma	6
Lung, bronchogenic carcinoma	6
Brain, glioma	3
Bladder, epithelioma	3
Larynx, squamous cell carcinoma	2
Pancreas, adenocarcinoma	2
Esophagus, squamous cell carcinoma	1
Jejunum, adenocarcinoma	1
Leukemia, chronic myelogenous	1
Lip, squamous cell carcinoma	1
Lymphosarcoma	1
Ovary, adenocarcinoma	1
Prostate, adenocarcinoma	1
Spinal cord, glioma	1
Tongue, squamous cell carcinoma	1
Bladder, epithelioma plus prostate, adenocarcinoma	1
Colon (2 lesions), adenocarcinoma	1
Colon, adenocarcinoma plus pancreas, adenocarcinoma	1
Colon, adenocarcinoma plus stomach, adenocarcinoma	1
Ovary, adenocarcinoma plus uterus, adenocarcinoma	1
Lip plus skin, multiple epitheliomas	1
Skin, multiple epitheliomas	1
Breast, adenocarcinoma plus lung, bronchogenic carcinoma plus uterus, adenocarcinoma	1
Colon (2 lesions), adenocarcinoma plus stomach, adenocarcinoma	1

not peculiar to this study alone. In smaller series, FOREMAN observed a rate of 47%, PEARSON and FITZGERALD, 31%; and WARREN and COYLE, 53%. It is difficult to conceive of any logical reason why this small neoplasm, which generally runs such an indolent course, should be associated with such a great frequency of second cancers. The most natural inclination is to attribute this observation to some artifact in case-finding that we and others have been unable to recognize. Yet, the carcinoid tumor has been found to have so may bizarre features that the possible significance of this association cannot be discarded.

It is of interest that we did not find the same relationship for carcinoid tumors of the rectum (CALDAROLA and associates). Of 147 patients found to have rectal carcinoids at the Mayo Clinic through 1960, only 11, or 7 %, had associated primary malignant neoplasms.

References

CALDAROLA, V. T., R. J. JACKMAN, C. G. MOERTEL, and M. B. DOCKERTY: Carcinoid tumors of the rectum. Amer. J. Surg. 107, 844 (1964).

FOREMAN, R. C.: Carcinoid tumors: Report of 38 cases. Ann. Surg. 136, 838 (1952).

MOERTEL, C. G., W. G. SAUER, M. B. DOCKERTY, and A. H. BAGGENSTOSS: Life history of the carcinoid tumor of the small intestine. Cancer (Philad.) 14, 901 (1961).

PEARSON, C. M., and P. J. FITZGERALD: Carcinoid tumors — a re-emphasis of their malignant nature: Review of 140 cases. Cancer (Philad.) 2, 1005 (1949).

WARREN, K. W., and E. B. COYLE: Carcinoid tumors of the gastrointestinal tract. Amer. J. Surg. 82, 372 (1951).

8. The Coexistence of Primary Lung Cancer and Other Primary Malignant Neoplasms

A solitary pulmonary lesion in a patient having a proved primary malignant neoplasm in another site presents a crucial problem in differential diagnosis. Many physicians feel that a heroic attempt to remove a pulmonary metastatic lesion by thoracic operation is an unjustifiably radical procedure. The possibility, however, that the presumed metastatic lesion may in fact be a second and potentially curable primary malignant lesion must always weigh heavily in the thoughts of even the most conservative. COTTON, as well as others, has presented differential factors in the diagnosis of primary and metastatic pulmonary neoplasms. He pointed out that a history of hemoptysis, the presence of cavitation, and a location in the upper part of the lung are all more characteristic of primary than of metastatic lung cancer. Whereas these features may help characterize a large series of patients, KELLY and LANGSTRON more recently have demonstrated that for the individual patient the clinical differentiation between these two situations is difficult, if not impossible.

The study by KELLY and LANGSTRON agreed with another by CAHAN in demonstrating that the presence of a second primary cancer in the lung is not an uncommon problem. In CAHAN's series of 2,502 cases of primary lung cancer seen at the Memorial Cancer Center, a total of 81 patients had proved primary cancers at some extrapulmonary site — a rate of occurrence of 3.2%. During the same period at the same institution, only 18 patients were found to have a solitary pulmonary metastatic neoplasm. From a study of 22 patients undergoing exploratory operation for solitary pulmonary lesions diagnosed preoperatively as metastatic, KELLY and LANGSTRON reported that 4 were found at thoracotomy to have unsuspected primary lung cancers. They concluded that in patients in whom there is reasonable evidence that a primary malignant lesion has been controlled, the presence of a discrete pulmonary lesion is an absolute indication for thoracotomy.

a) Selection of Cases

All the patients whose cases are included in our study had a lung cancer plus another unequivocally malignant neoplasm verified at this clinic's laboratories during the period of this study. Cases in which the lung cancer had been diagnosed by cytologic examination of the sputum alone were excluded.

The fact that the lung is a common site for almost all types of metastatic malignant lesions compounds the difficulty of establishing a pulmonary lesion as a true second primary cancer. Several cases initially diagnosed as presenting second primary cancers in the lung were discarded from the present study because after review of the pathologic material doubt existed as to whether the pulmonary lesion was actually a primary lesion. Some of these discarded cases possibly represented true but unconfirmable primary cancers.

b) Observations

During the 10-year period included in this study, a total of 1,588 patients at the Mayo Clinic had the diagnosis of primary cancer of the lung, bronchus, or pleura confirmed by laboratory examination of specimens obtained at bronchoscopy, thoracotomy, or autopsy. Of this group a total of 65 patients, or 4.1%, were found to have one or more other primary malignant neoplasms. Of these patients 59 were male and 6 were female.

In 27 cases the lesions were diagnosed simultaneously; in 8 cases diagnosis of the pulmonary lesion preceded the diagnosis of the other neoplasm by periods of 1 to 5 years; and in 30 cases the diagnosis of the pulmonary lesion followed the diagnosis of the other neoplasm by periods of 1 to 29 years (average 9.6 years).

In 24 cases both lesions were diagnosed at operation only; in 8 cases both lesions

Table 18. *Specific Types and Locations of Associated Primary Malignant Neoplasms Found in Patients With Primary Lung Cancer*

Types and locations	Cases	Types and locations	Cases
Carcinoma of		Carcinoma of	
Skin or lips	13	Pancreas and skin	1
Colon or rectum	9	Prostate and thyroid	1
Prostate	9	Leukemia or lymphoma	4
Bladder	5	Carcinoid (multiple) of ileum	2
Oral cavity	4	Fibrosarcoma	1
Breast	2	Malignant melanoma	1
Kidney	2	Seminoma	1
Larynx	2	Multiple myeloma and	
Ovary	1	epithelioma of skin	1
Pancreas	1	Fibrosarcoma; epithelioma	
Stomach	1	(multiple) of lips and skin;	
Thyroid	1	adenocarcinoma of parotid	1
Lip and prostate	1		
Mouth and skin	1		

were diagnosed at autopsy only; and in 33 cases one or more lesions were diagnosed both at operation and at autopsy.

The distribution of the specific types of second primary cancers, shown in Table 18, does not seem significantly different from that to be expected in a random selection of patients of comparable age and sex with single malignant neoplasms. It is of interest that 37 of CAHAN's series of 81 patients, or 46%, were found to have their second primary lesions involving the oral cavity or larynx. He postulated that this association could represent the effect of a common etiologic agent in cancers of the oral cavity, larynx, and lung. In our study, only 7 of 65 patients, or 11%, had second primary lesions in these locations. Since the vast majority of patients with lung cancer are males in the older age groups, this does not seem a disproportionate representation of cancers of the oral cavity and larynx.

Of incidental interest is the fact that at autopsy a primary carcinoma of the lung was found that had metastasized to a primary cancer of the kidney (Fig. 7). It appears that instances in which one malignant neoplasm is found to have

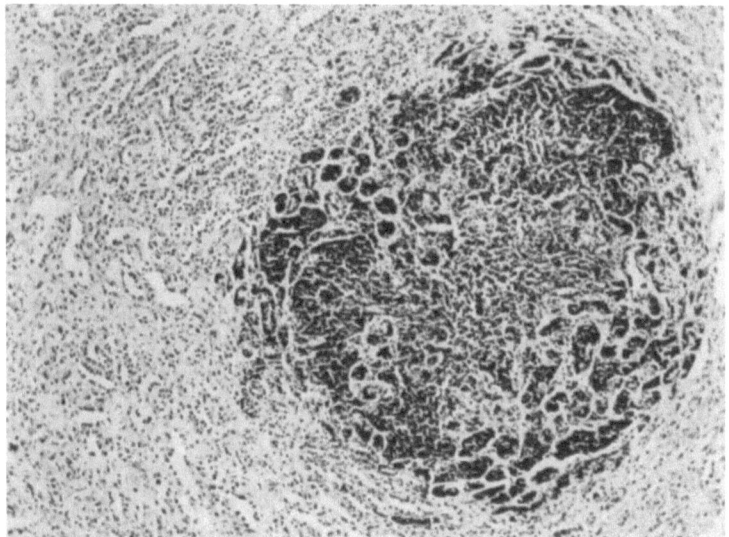

Fig. 7. Bronchogenic carcinoma, small cell type, metastatic to adenocarcinoma, hypernephroma type, of the kidney. (Hematoxylin and eosin; ×75.)

metastasized to a second independent malignant neoplasm are exceedingly rare; when GORE and BARR reviewed the literature in 1958 they could find only 21 cases, including the 2 which they reported. It is of interest that in 15 of these 21 cases, as well as in that reported here, the recipient cancer was a hypernephroma.

c) Comment

The evidence presented here as well as in the other works cited seems to establish definitely that the occurrence of an independent primary lung cancer in a patient with known malignant neoplastic disease at another site is not uncommon. Therefore no solitary pulmonary lesion in a patient with a previously diagnosed cancer may be simply assumed to be metastatic without positive laboratory confirmation. The present-day risk of thoracotomy in an otherwise doomed patient should be inconsequential when weighed against the possible tragedy of ignoring a potentially curable lung cancer on the grounds that it may be a solitary metastatic lesion. Indeed, even if the lesion should prove to be metastatic, hope may be found in CAHAN's records of many patients with surprisingly long survival and no evidence of metastasis to other sites following excision of a solitary metastatic pulmonary lesion. Our series serves as further evidence supporting the conclusion of KELLY and LANGSTRON that in cases affording reasonable evidence that a primary malignant lesion elsewhere has been controlled, the presence of a discrete pulmonary lesion is an absolute indication for thoracotomy.

References

CAHAN, W. G.: Lung cancer associated with cancer primary in other sites. Amer. J. Surg. **89**, 494 (1955).

COTTON, B. H.: Differential diagnosis of primary and metastatic malignancy of the lung. Amer. J. Surg. **54**, 173 (1941).

GORE, IRA, and RICHARD BARR: Metastasis of cancer to cancer. A. M. A. Arch. Path. **66**, 293 (1958).

KELLY, C. R., and H. T. LANGSTRON: The treatment of metastatic pulmonary malignancy. J. thorac. Surg. **31**, 298 (1956).

Summary

At this time there is no acceptable evidence either in this presentation or in the literature that the patterns of occurrence of multiple primary malignant neoplasms of different organs or tissues are governed by anything more than coincidence. The frequency of occurrence of specific types of second primary cancers is probably largely determined by the age of the patient at the time of diagnosis of the initial cancer and the expected longevity after treatment of the initial lesion. There is no factual basis at present for assuming that the existence of any one malignant neoplasm, with the possible exception of the carcinoid tumor of the small intestine, implies any systemic carcinogenic influence or that it implies any increased susceptibility of any other organ or organ system to future malignant disease.

It is possible that in some cases therapeutic procedures employed in treatment of a specific malignant neoplasm may exert a carcinogenic influence on other organs or tissues. This seems to be well established in cases in which lymphangiosarcoma develops at the site of postmastectomy lymphedema. There is also evidence for believing that ionizing radiation as used in cancer therapy may have a carcinogenic or leukemogenic effect; this is particularly true when large doses of ^{131}I are used for treating thyroid cancer.

In an attempt to determine whether hereditofamilial influences are significant in patients with multiple primary cancers of different organs or tissues, the family histories of malignant disease given by the patients in this series were studied in relation to those given by comparable groups of patients with single cancers and of patients with no evidence of malignant disease. When compared with these two control groups, patients with multiple primary cancers were found to have an increased family incidence of malignant disease. This increase was most prominent in family members of the younger age groups. This was a retrospective study, however, and the results must be interpreted with caution.

There is no evidence that a patient's ABO blood group is in any way related to a tendency to multiple cancer formation.

Probably the most important point to be emphasized in this section is the simple fact that second primary cancers can and do develop in different organs and tissues.

These lesions may appear either simultaneously with another primary cancer or after successful treatment of an initial primary cancer. Usually there is no reliable clinical means of distinguishing a second primary lesion from a solitary metastatic lesion. In these cases definitive diagnosis must be made by exploration, biopsy, and pathologic examination.

C. Multiple Primary Malignant Neoplasms of Multicentric Origin
1. Introductory Comments

Multicentric neoplastic change must be anticipated when a common tissue, presumably endowed with a common susceptibility to malignant disease, is exposed to a common carcinogenic influence. Both of these criteria — a common tissue and exposure to common carcinogenic influence — must be met before true multicentric malignant change will take place. We will demonstrate in this section that multicentric carcinoma of the common squamous epithelium of the oral cavity, pharynx, and larynx occurs quite frequently. However, it has been demonstrated in the previous section and will be amplified in this one that this tendency to multicentricity does not extend to the contiguous columnar epithelium of the trachea and bronchi, although both epithelial surfaces are exposed to the same presumably carcinogenic respiratory irritants. Similarly, multicentric epitheliomas of the skin are exceedingly common in the patient whose occupation requires prolonged exposure of the skin to sun and wind. These lesions, however, are distinctly limited to the exposed surfaces of the skin; the unexposed skin surfaces, although they are of the same type of tissue, are not exposed to the same carcinogenic influence.

The major types of multicentric cancer and their frequency of occurrence are presented in Table 19. These will be discussed individually in the subsequent sections.

Table 19. *Incidence of Multicentricity in Epithelial Carcinomas*

Location	Patients	Multicentric lesions, %
In same organ or tissue		
Skin (COOPER, PHILLIPS)	(Literature)	6 to 42
Oral cavity	732	8.7
Lips	1,300	6.3
Stomach	1,835	2.2
Small intestine: carcinoids	209	29
Large intestine	6,012	4.3
Bladder	112	19.0
Vulva and vagina	137	5.8
Brain and spinal cord: glioma	305	4.9
In bilaterally paired organs		
Breasts	2,945	4.0
Testes	226	2.2

References

COOPER, Z. K.: A study of 106 cases of multiple primary skin cancer. Surg. Clin. N. Amer. Oct., 1022 (1944).

PHILLIPS, CHARLES: Multiple skin cancer: A statistical and pathologic study. Sth. med. J. (Bgham, Ala.) **35**, 583 (1942).

2. Multicentric Epitheliomas of the Skin

The marked tendency to multicentricity exhibited by epitheliomas of the skin is obvious to all who have had even casual experience with this condition. The reported incidence of proved multiple simultaneous lesions varies from 6 % (Cooper) to 16 % (Phillips). The incidence of proved multiple lesions is probably far less than the true incidence since many lesions are commonly treated by cautery without biopsy. That this tendency to multicentricity is frequently related to exposure to the sun has been demonstrated by Cooper, who followed for $2^1/_2$ years the course of 55 patients who had cancers of the skin and outdoor occupations. During this short time, new skin cancers developed in 23 patients (41.8 %). MacDonald found that of 566 patients with multiple skin cancers, 431 had all lesions confined to exposed areas.

Studies of cancer of the skin have provided evidence that lesions seen clinically as single neoplasms frequently have their origin from multiple areas of neoplastic change. This was first demonstrated by Molesworth in 1927. Later detailed studies by Willis again demonstrated the multicentric origin of skin cancer and led him to make the following observations: "It is, I think, very doubtful if an epidermal growth ever takes origin from a single minute focus at a single moment of time.... . The still prevalent view that tumors usually arise at a single point in time from a single small focus is false."

It seemed likely that contiguous exposed squamous epithelium of the lips would be affected by multicentric carcinomas of the skin. Of the 5,000 patients with carcinomas of the skin seen at the Mayo Clinic during the 10-year period of this study, a total of 172 (3.4 %) were found to have discrete squamous cell epitheliomas of the lips also.

References

Cooper, Z. K.: A study of 106 cases of multiple primary skin cancer. Surg. Clin. N. Amer. Oct., 1022 (1944).

MacDonald, Eleanor J.: Occurrence of multiple primary cancers in a population of 200,000. Acta Un. int. Cancr. 16, 1702 (1960).

Molesworth, E. H.: Rodent ulcer. Med. J. Aust. 1, 878 (1927).

Phillips, Charles: Multiple skin cancer: A statistical and pathologic study. Sth. med. J. (Bgham, Ala.) 35, 583 (1942).

Willis, R. A.: Further studies on the mode of origin of carcinomas of the skin. Cancer Res. 5, 469 (1945).

3. Multicentric Carcinomas of the Oral Cavity

Many of the basic observations underlying the concept of multicentric origin of epithelial malignancy have been made in the study of carcinoma of the oral cavity. Here the lesions are readily accessible to direct observations, and the relationship of possible carcinogenic influences and premalignant lesions to the ensuing carcinoma is frequently quite convincing.

Sarasin was the first to publish a detailed study of this problem when in 1933 he presented 30 cases of nonsimultaneous multiple epitheliomas of the oral cavity. Later in that same year, after a statistical study of 1,548 cases of carcinoma of the buccal cavity (including the lips), LUND concluded that the incidence of second primary lesions in the buccal cavity was approximately 15 times greater than that expected by chance alone. In 1946 after a study of 80 patients with intraoral carcinoma, SLAUGHTER found that 14 patients, or 18 %, had grossly apparent multi-centric lesions. In 1952 BYARS and ANDERSON reviewed 166 cases of cancer of the oral cavity; after excluding contiguous lesions and multicentric lesions in a single area of leukoplakia, they still found that 20 patients, or 12 %, had multiple oral cancers. In 1957 WILKINS and VOGLER reported that of 81 patients with gingival cancer, a total of 17, or 21 %, had multiple lesions of the oral cavity. Evidence that this tendency to multicentricity may also extend to include the epithelium of the pharynx, larynx, and esophagus has been presented in studies of SCHEEL, ENGEL-BRETH-HOLM, VIDEBAEK, and MOUNIER-KUHN and associates.

a) Selection of Cases

The pathologic findings were reviewed in all cases of carcinoma of the oral cavity proved by examination of surgical specimens. The clinical, surgical, and pathologic records were reviewed in all cases in which two or more specimens had been submitted and proved malignant by pathologic examination. Cases were included in the present study as multiple simultaneous carcinomas if the patient had two or more discrete lesions clearly separated by normal mucosa. Cases were included as multiple nonsimultaneous cancers only if the most recent lesion was clearly separated from the site of excision of the initial lesion, regardless of the time inter-vening between diagnoses of the two lesions. All cases were discarded in which any reasonable doubt existed that one of the lesions may have represented a recurrence, local extension, or metastasis from a single primary focus.

b) Observations

During the 10-year period of this study, a total of 732 patients (578 males, 154 females) were found at the Mayo Clinic to have pathologically confirmed squamous cell carcinomas of the oral cavity, that is, fauces, palate, tongue, gingivae, and buccal surfaces. Of this group, a total of 64 patients (55 males, 9 females) were demonstrated to have multiple discrete carcinomas of the oral cavity — a rate of occurrence of 8.7%. All lesions were squamous cell carcinomas. Of the 64 patients, 21 had simultaneous lesions and 43 had lesions occurring at intervals ranging from 1 to 25 years, the average interval being 7.1 years.

The frequency of occurrence of leukoplakia in association with multicentric oral cancer was noted by SARASIN as 67 % in the patients of his study. WILKINS and VOGLER reported the incidence of associated leukoplakia in their patients with multiple oral cancers to be 79 %, whereas it was only 40 % in their entire series of patients with gingival cancer. A comparably high association of this presumed premalignant condition also was noted in this study — 48 of the 64 patients in this series were observed to have leukoplakia demonstrated by either clinical or patho-logic examination.

SARASIN also suggested syphilis and tobacco as possible etiologic factors in the patients in his series (Fig. 8). In the present study, the histories or serologic studies for five patients, or 7.8 %, gave evidence of previous syphilitic infection. A definite history of the use of, or abstinence from, tobacco was obtained from 49 of the male patients in this study. Of this group, 46, or 94 %, were using or had used tobacco in some form. It is of interest that 22, or 48 %, of those using tobacco either smoked

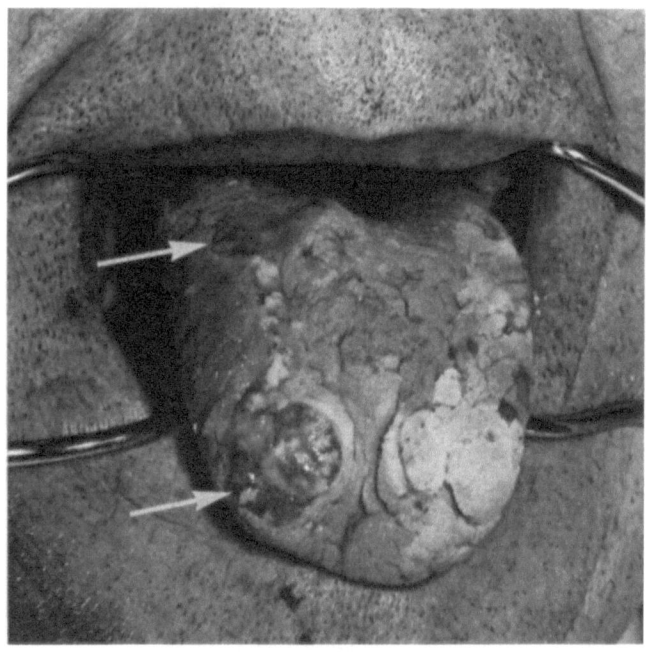

Fig. 8. Multiple carcinomas on a tongue with extensive leukoplakia. The results of serologic tests were positive (positive Kline, Kahn, Hinton, and Kolmer tests), and the patient gave a history of heavy smoking

cigars or chewed, thus repeatedly bathing the mouth in tobacco juices. This relationship was brought out strikingly in one elderly gentleman, who had chewed for his entire adult life and habitually pouched his chaw in his right cheek. When seen at this clinic, the entire right buccal surface, and only the right buccal surface, was the site of extensive leukoplakia and two discrete squamous cell carcinomas. WILKINS and VOGLER reported a similar disproportion in tobacco habits in their series of patients with gingival cancer — 57 % of all their male patients who used tobacco either chewed tobacco cuttings or used snuff. It would be presumptuous to state that the evidence presented in this study and the others quoted constitutes statistically valid proof that tobacco is an etiologic factor in the production of oral cancer; however, the inference is so strong that it can hardly be ignored. It is the responsibility of the physician to interdict firmly the use of tobacco in any form by all patients treated for oral cancer or with premalignant leukoplakia.

That the tendency to multicentricity in oral carcinoma is not limited to the oral cavity alone but extends to the contiguous squamous cell mucous membrane is evidenced by the fact that an additional 55 patients with oral cancer had associated epitheliomas of the lips, pharynx, larynx, or esophagus. The overall occurrence rate of multicentric cancer for the 732 patients in this group is thus raised to 16.4 %.

c) Comment

Whereas the occurrence of grossly apparent multicentric lesions in this series and in the literature is substantial, still more impressive is the histologic study of SLAUGHTER. By careful examination of 14 operative specimens of coral carcinoma, he found that 13 of the 14 showed definite microscopic evidence of multicentricity. He further concluded that many so-called recurrences may in reality be new foci of cancer arising in the peripheral field of a previously treated epithelioma.

LUND stated that in the patient with known oral cancer, even when no premalignant lesion such as leukoplakia is visible, the entire buccal mucosa must be considered to be in a premalignant condition. With this possibility in mind, any physician who assumes the responsibility of caring for these patients also must assume the responsibility of insisting on frequent and regular follow-up examinations. In addition, SARASIN has suggested the following steps as positive measures in preventing the development of a second cancer which might well be re-emphasized here: (1) eradicate leukoplakia, (2) stop the use of tobacco, (3) eliminate alveolar-dental infection, and (4) correct defective dental prosthetic devices.

Summary

When oral cancer develops, all of the contiguous squamous mucous membrane must be considered as highly susceptible to future malignant change. It is the responsibility of the physician to insist on frequent and regular follow-up examinations so that any second lesion may be detected and treated in its early stages. It is also his responsibility to initiate appropriate prophylactic measures to eliminate any possible sources of carcinogenic irritation to these regions.

References

BYARS, L. T., and R. ANDERSON: Multiple cancers of oral cavity. Amer. Surg. 18, 386 (1952).

ENGELBRETH-HOLM, J.: Om multiple carcinomer i mundsvaelgoesophagus. Nord. Med. 16, 3171 (1942).

LUND, C. C.: Second primary cancer in cases of cancer of buccal mucosa: Mathematical study of susceptibility to cancer. New Engl. J. Med. 209, 1144 (1933).

MOUNIER-KUHN, P., J. GAILLARD, J. P. REBATTU, and B. JAKUBOWICZ: Statistique des cancers multiples à la clinique oto-rhino-laryngologique de Lyon de 1950 à 1962. Lyon méd. 212, 1389 (1964).

SARASIN, R.: Les manifestations successives des épithéliomas des muqueuses de la cavité buccale: Sont elles des récidives vaies ou résultent-elles de nouvelles cancérisations? Radiophys. et radiothérapie 3, 33 (1933).

SCHEEL, AXEL: Multiple kancere i munnhule — svelg — spiserør. Nord. Med. 15, 2165 (1942).

SLAUGHTER, D. P.: Multicentric origin of intraoral carcinoma. Surgery 20, 133 (1946).

VIDEBAEK, A.: Solitary and multiple carcinomas of upper alimentary tract; their location, age, and sex incidence and correlation with Plummer-Vinson syndrome. Acta radiol. (Stockh.) 25, 339 (1944).

WILKINS, S. A., JR., and W. R. VOGLER: Cancer of the gingiva. Surg. Gynec. Obstet. 105, 145 (1957).

4. Multicentric Epitheliomas of the Lips

Despite the smaller surface area involved, multicentric epitheliomas of the lips were observed only slightly less frequently than multicentric epitheliomas of the oral cavity. During the 10-year period of this study a total of 1,300 patients were seen at the Mayo Clinic with pathologically proved epitheliomas of the lips. Among these patients were 82 who had multicentric lesions, a rate of occurrence of 6.3%. Fifty-three patients had simultaneous and 29 had interval lesions. Both multiple and single lesions showed a strong predilection for the lower rather than the upper lip.

As early as 1921 microscopic multicentricity of origin of carcinoma of the lip was demonstrated by WARWICK. Since the squamous epithelium of the lips is contiguous with both the skin and the mucous membrane of the upper part of the digestive and respiratory tracts, the occurrence of multicentric epitheliomas of the lips would be expected with epitheliomas of both of these surfaces. This was found to be the case, as 131 of the 1,300 patients with epitheliomas of the lips also had epitheliomas of the skin, an occurrence rate of 10.1%. Similar findings have been recorded by EINHORN and JAKOBSSON, who documented 82 patients with second primary carinomas of the skin among 1,675 with carcinoma of the lip. Forty-five of our patients also had epitheliomas of the oral cavity, pharynx, larynx, or esophagus — an occurrence rate of 3.5%.

That the lesions in these patients are in truth multicentric manifestations of a common carcinogenic tendency rather than coincidental occurrences is evidenced by the fact that of the 285 patients in this series who had an epithelioma of the lip and a second primary lesion, 235 (82.5%) had a second lesion which involved the same squamous epithelium or contiguous squamous epithelium of the upper aerodigestive tract or of the skin.

References

EINHORN, J., and P. JAKOBSSON: Multiple primary malignant tumors. Cancer (Philad.) **17**, 1437 (1964).

WARWICK, MARGARET: Model of carcinoma of the lip reconstructed from serial section. J. Amer. med. Ass. **82**, 1119 (1924).

5. Multicentric Epitheliomas Involving the Larynx, Pharynx, and Esophagus

Of 1,100 patients with squamous cell carcinoma of the larynx proved at operation during the 10 years covered by this study, a total of 18 (1.6%) were found to have two discrete lesions. For the most part these patients had a single lesion on each vocal cord. Eleven patients had simultaneous lesions, and seven had interval lesions. In addition to these, 22 patients with carcinoma of the larynx had associated squamous cell carcinomas involving the lips, oral cavity, pharynx, or esophagus. Overall then, 40 of the 1,100 patients with carcinoma of the larynx (3.6%) had multicentric lesions of the larynx or contiguous squamous epithelium.

Similar tendencies to multicentric lesions were found in patients with squamous cell carcinomas of the pharynx and esophagus. Eleven (7%) of 158 patients with squamous cell carcinoma of the pharynx and 10 (2.4%) of 421 patients with squamous cell carcinoma of the esophagus also had associated squamous cell lesions of contiguous epithelium. These findings are closely similar to those of MOUNIER-KUHN and associates. Of 2,522 patients with carcinoma of the upper aerodigestive tract, 121 (4.8%) were found to have multicentric lesions. They found only 19 cases (0.8%) of neoplasms primary to other sites.

It is worthy of note that of 1,258 patients with carcinomas of the pharynx or larynx in this study, only 2 were found to have bronchogenic carcinomas. This also corresponds to the findings of Mounier-Kuhn and associates: two cancers of the tracheobronchial tree among 2,522 patients with carcinomas of the upper aerodigestive tract. In spite of speculations of some authors, the combination of bronchogenic and laryngeal or pharyngeal carcinomas in the same patient cannot be construed by currently available evidence as anything more than coincidence.

Reference

Mounier-Kuhn, P., J. Gaillard, J. P. Rebattu, and B. Jakubowicz: Statistique des cancers multiples à la clinique oto-rhino-laryngologique de Lyon de 1950 à 1962. Lyon méd. 212, 1389 (1964).

6. Multicentric Adenocarcinomas of the Stomach

In 1855, what was probably the first recorded case of multiple gastric cancers was presented by Barth before the Anatomical Society of Paris. Such cases remained rare in subsequent years, so that Warren and Gates, in 1932, could add only 34 recorded cases of multiple primary malignant gastric neoplasms from the world literature. In 1943, Brindley and associates first drew attention to the relative frequency of multiple cancers of the stomach by reporting 23 cases seen at the Mayo Clinic during a single decade. A review of the world literature to date reveals a total of 147 published cases of multiple gastric malignant neoplasms exclusive of the cases included in this report. The incidence of this phenomenon was reported by the authors listed in Table 20.

Table 20. *Reported Incidence of Multiple Gastric Cancers*

Authors	Total cases of gastric cancer	Cases of multiple gross gastric cancers	Incidence, %
Albrecht	1,206	10	0.83
Brindley *et al.*	1,184	23	1.94
Brown and Moots	500	5	1.00
Oota and Tanaka	354	5	1.40
Goriainowa and Schabad	334	2	0.60
MacDonald	293	7	2.39
Warren	243	0	0.00
Moore and Morton	163	1	0.61
Collins and Gall	117	4	3.42

Of major significance is the study of Collins and Gall. Although gross examination revealed only four multiple lesions among their 117 cases of gastric carcinoma, careful microscopic studies demonstrated zones of carcinoma in situ distinctly separate from the main lesions in an additional 22 cases. Their overall incidence of multiple malignant gastric lesions thus was increased to 22%.

a) Present Study

The pathologic findings were reviewed in all cases of gastric cancer diagnosed at the time of gastrectomy or from autopsy specimens seen at the Mayo Clinic in the 10-year period ending January 1, 1954. Cases in which two or more lesions were present were accepted as examples of multiple malignant neoplasms only if they met the following three criteria: (1) each lesion must be of pathologically proved malignancy; (2) all lesions must be separated distinctly by microscopically normal gastric wall; (3) the possibility that one of the lesions represents a local extension or metastatic tumor must be ruled out beyond any reasonable doubt.

Only tumors of unequivocal malignancy were included in this study. Lesions consisting only of low-grade carcinoma in situ in adenomatous polyps were not included, because this diagnosis is frequently somewhat subjective and because the true malignancy of these lesions is still a subject of debate. Microscopic examination of the intervening gastric wall was an essential step in proving the multiplicity of lesions, since lesions presumed to be multiple on gross examination in several cases were found by histologic examination to be continuous through extensive submucosal communications.

b) Results

Multiple Simultaneous Gastric Cancers. — By use of the criteria just listed, a total of 40 cases were confirmed as representing multiple simultaneous gastric cancers among the 1,835 gastric cancers proved at gastrectomy or autopsy during the period of this study. A total of 34 patients were men and 6 were women; the lesions were verified at gastrectomy in 37 cases and at autopsy in 3. The average age at diagnosis in the men was 62 years, whereas it was 54 years in the women. The range of age was from 40 to 81 years.

The incidence of multiple gastric cancers in this series is given in Table 21. A total of 38 patients had multiple adenocarcinomas. Of these, 29 patients had two lesions and 9 had three lesions; 26 of these patients had tumors of different grades of malignancy and 12 had tumors of the same grade (Fig. 9). In addition to the 38 patients who had multiple adenocarcinomas, 1 patient had two independent leiomyosarcomas and 1 had simultaneous adenocarcinoma and leiomyosarcoma.

Table 21. *Incidence of Multiple Simultaneous Gastric Cancers in a 10-Year Period at the Mayo Clinic*

	Total cases of gastric cancer	Cases of multiple gross gastric cancers	Incidence, %
MEN	1,401	34	2.42
WOMEN	434	6	1.38
Total	1,835	40	2.18

Multiple Nonsimultaneous Gastric Cancers. — Reports of independent cancers in the gastric remnant after apparently successful subtotal gastrectomy for a previous malignant tumor are extremely few. By reviewing the literature prior to 1964, Irons was able to cull only 17 cases which seemed well documented and probably represented independent lesions. This rarity may be actual or it may be only apparent because of the practical difficulties encountered in authenticating such cases.

The evidence presented in the two cases to follow appears to establish them as true examples of independent nonsimultaneous gastric carcinomas. How many other such lesions have occurred under the guise of recurrence is only conjectural.

Case 1. — A 64-year-old man came to the Mayo Clinic in January 1934 because of recurrent postprandial epigastric distress, occasional vomiting, and progressive loss of weight for 2½ years. Results of physical examination were not remarkable, but a gastric roentgenogram showed ulceration on the lesser curvature. Subtotal gastric resection was performed. Pathologic examination revealed a grade 3 ulcerative adenocarcinoma of the lesser curvature, with no evidence of local extension or nodal involvement (Fig. 10A).

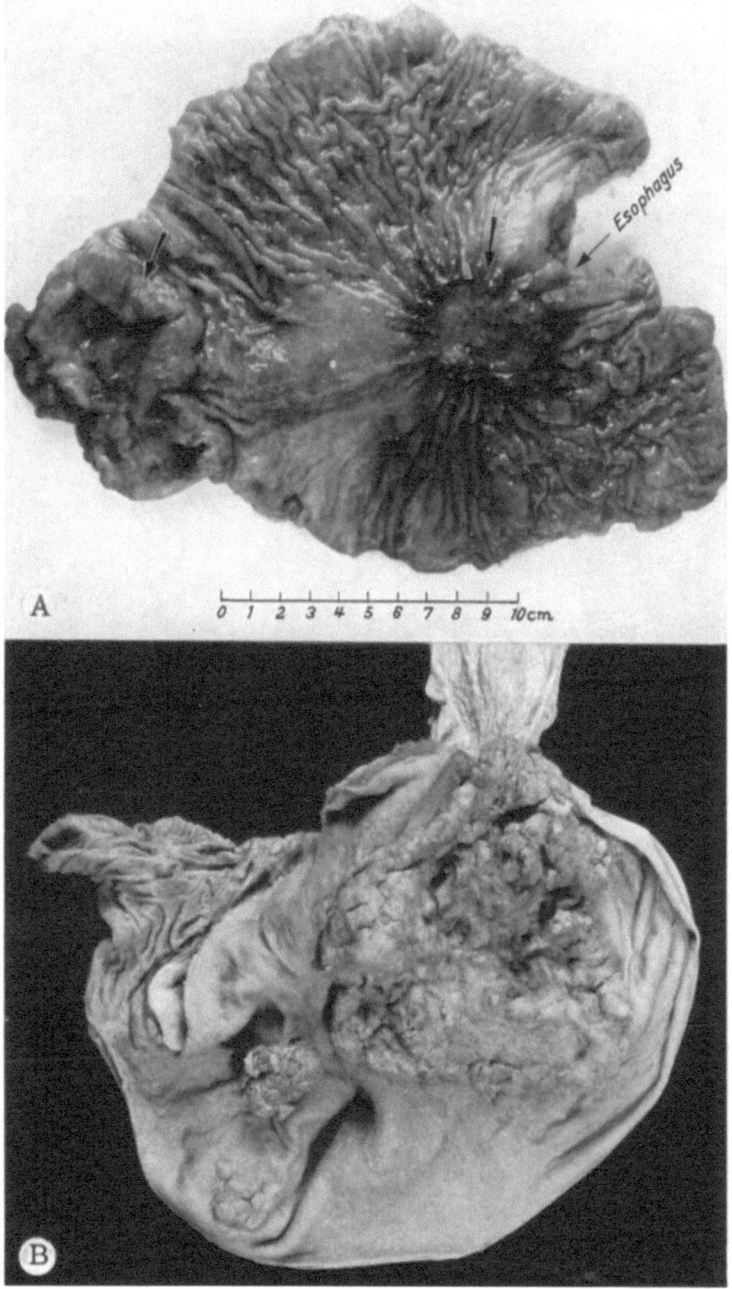

Fig. 9. *A*, Two simultaneous ulcerating grade 3 adenocarcinomas of the stomach (surgical specimen). *B*, Three simultaneous fungating grade 1, grade 2, and grade 4 adenocarcinomas of the stomach (autopsy specimen)

The patient then remained entirely well until 8¹/₂ years later, when he noted the onset of epigastric pain, anorexia, occasional vomiting, and loss of weight. He returned to this clinic in October 1944, almost 11 years after his initial operation, and a second gastrectomy was performed. Pathologic examination at this time revealed a grade 4 polypoid and ulcerating scirrhous adenocarcinoma of the gastric remnant (Fig. 10 B). There was no evidence

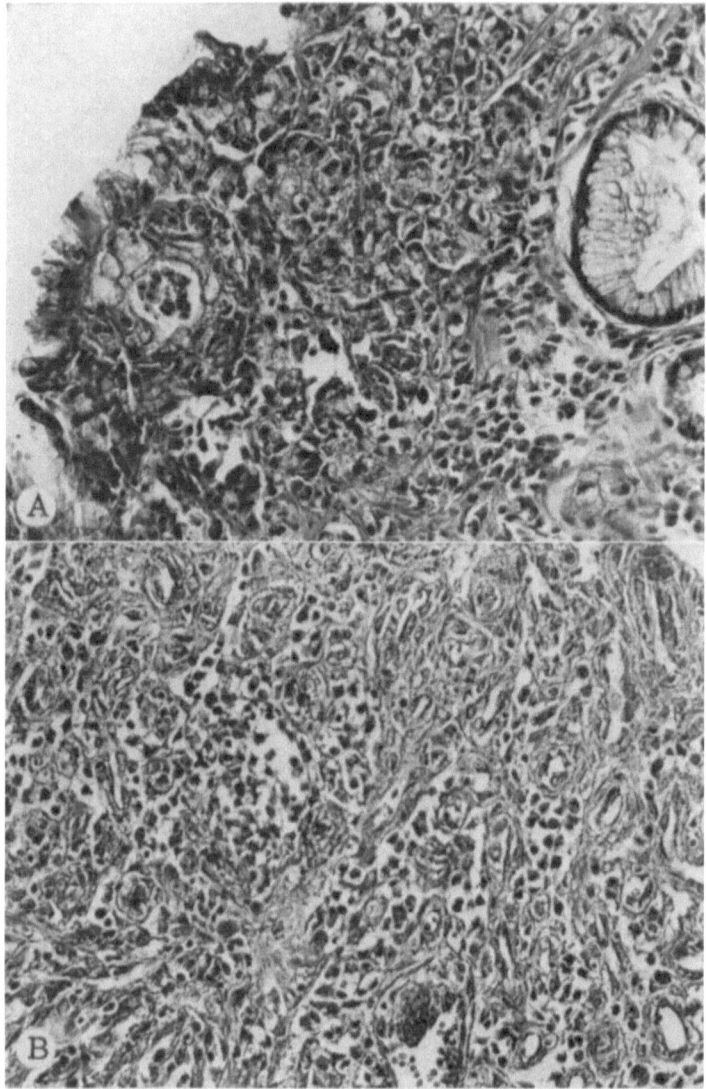

Fig. 10 (case 1). *A,* Superficial grade 3 adenocarcinoma found at subtotal gastrectomy in 1934. *B,* Grade 4 scirrhous adenocarcinoma found in the gastric remnant in 1944. (Hematoxylin and eosin; ×265.)

of distant metastasis, but three adjacent lymph nodes were involved. The patient died of respiratory complications on the twenty-third postoperative day. Autopsy was not performed.

The long symptom-free interval combined with the high grade of the malignancy of the second lesion makes it probable that the second carcinoma represented an entirely new lesion rather than a recurrent tumor.

Case 2. — A 32-year-old man came to the Mayo Clinic in August 1939 because of a 4-year history of burning epigastric pain occurring 2 hours after meals. A gastric roentgenogram showed an ulcer on the lesser curvature. Subtotal gastrectomy was performed. Pathologic examination showed an ulcerating grade 4 mucous adenocarcinoma just above the pylorus (Fig. 11 *A*).

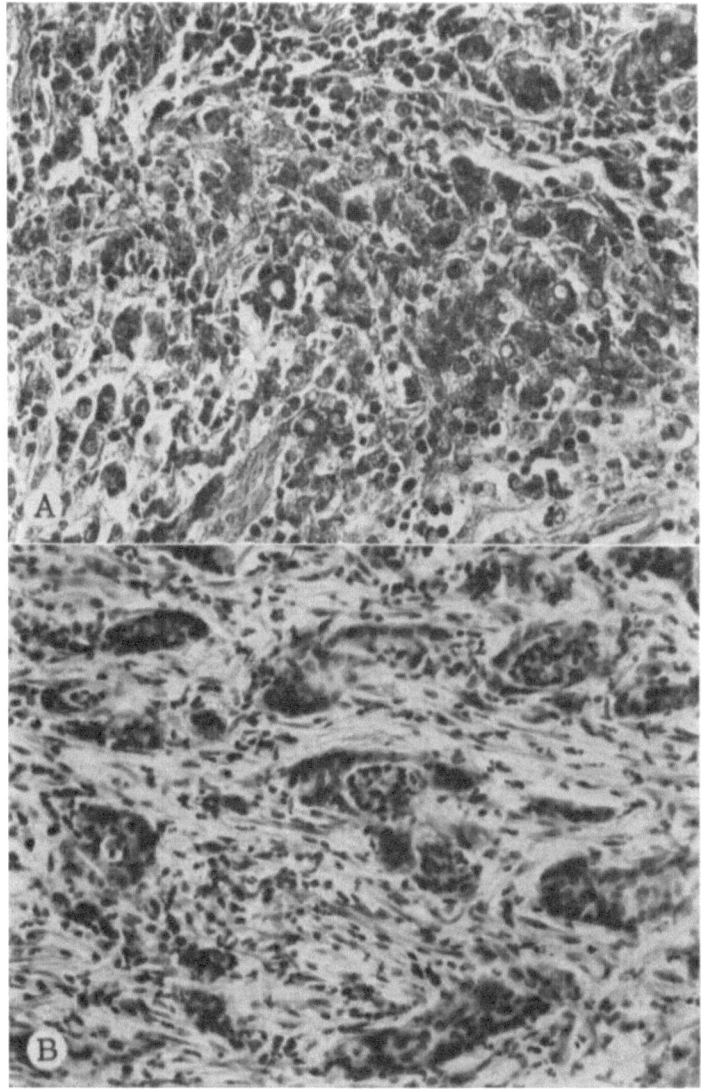

Fig. 11 (case 2). *A*, Grade 4 mucous adenocarcinoma found at subtotal gastrectomy in 1939. *B*, Grade 3 scirrhous adenocarcinoma found in the gastric remnant in 1953. (Hematoxylin and eosin; ×265.)

The patient then remained free of symptoms for 14 years. Gastric roentgenograms in 1940 and 1951 were negative. In September 1953 he returned complaining of epigastric distress, occasional vomiting, weakness, and loss of weight. A roentgenogram showed an ulcerating lesion in the gastric remnant. Abdominal exploration revealed an inoperable lesion of the stomach invading the transverse colon and jejunum. There was no evidence of distant metastasis. Biopsy disclosed a grade 3 scirrhous carcinoma distinctly different from the earlier lesion (Fig. 11 *B*). The patient died at home 2 months later.

The 14-year symptom-free and roentgenologically negative interval in this case, plus the distinctly different histopathologic appearance of the two lesions, is strongly in favor of their being two independent carcinomas.

Association of Multiple Gastric Cancers With Other Conditions. 1. Pernicious Anemia. — Three of these 42 patients had pernicious anemia, either diagnosed previously and being treated or discovered at the time of diagnosis of the multiple gastric cancers. The association of gastric carcinoma and pernicious anemia has been reviewed by SCHELL and co-workers. In a study of 48 patients with both pernicious anemia and carcinoma of the stomach, they found that 13 (27 %) had multiple gastric tumors. When this is compared with the incidence of 2.2 % found in this study, it appears that the incidence of multiple gastric cancers is approximately 12 times as frequent in patients who have pernicious anemia and cancer of the stomach as it is in an overall series of patients with gastric cancer.

2. Gastric Polyposis. — Four of the patients in the present study had associated gastric polyposis. During the 10-year period of this study, a total of 21 patients seen at this clinic were proved to have combined gastric polyposis and gastric carcinoma. The four patients just mentioned represent a 19 % incidence of multiple gastric malignant tumors in this group of 21 patients. An additional five patients (24 %) had one or more polyps showing in situ carcinomatous changes associated with a single unequivocally malignant neoplasm. As mentioned previously, cases like these were not considered in the present study.

c) Comment

In the case of gastric cancer, the grossly uninvolved gastric mucosa presumably has been exposed to the same carcinogenic influences that incited the initial neoplasm, be they inflammation, ingested carcinogens, or other entities as yet unknown.

It is reasonable to assume that at least a significant proportion of gastric cancers would present multicentric zones of malignant change at some stage in their development. The fact that 2.2 % of the gastric cancers in our series were grossly multicentric and that 22 % in the series of COLLINS and GALL were microscopically multicentric appears to give ample evidence for this assumption.

That this concept of multicentric gastric cancer may be of more than didactic importance has been expressed by TEPERSON and associates, who said that, "the incidence of multiple lesions is an added straw in the wind of prevailing opinion that total gastrectomy is a more nearly ideal procedure for carcinoma of the stomach than is subtotal gastrectomy." WALTERS and co-workers reported that 40 of 120 patients followed after Billroth I resection probably had recurrence in or around the remaining part of the stomach. A least a small proportion of these patients actually may have had a new lesion in the gastric remnant indistinguishable from a recurrent tumor.

It is not the purpose of this report to advocate total gastrectomy for all patients who have gastric cancer, as it is obvious that many factors must be considered in addition to the multicentricity of gastric malignant tumors. There can be no doubt, however, that the frequency of multiple gastric cancers must be considered in any discussion of the relative merits of total versus subtotal gastrectomy. The physician must be especially aware of the great predilection to multiplicity of gastric cancer in patient who have gastric polyposis or pernicious anemia.

References

ALBRECHT, P.: Über die Multiplizität primärer maligner Geschwülste. Oncologia (Basel) **5**, 12 (1952).

BARTH: (Abstract of presentation). Bull. Soc. anat. Paris. **30**, 1 (1855).

BRINDLEY, G. V., JR., M. B. DOCKERTY, and H. K. GRAY: Multiple carcinomas of the stomach: Report of case. Proc. Mayo Clin. **18**, 193 (1943).

BROWN, C. H., and M. F. MOOTS: Multiple gastric carcinoma. Gastroenterology **26**, 846 (1954).

COLLINS, W. T., and E. A. GALL: Gastric carcinoma: A multicentric lesion. Cancer (Philad.) **5**, 62 (1952).

GORIAINOWA, R. W., and L. M. SCHABAD: Zur Frage der multiplen primären Geschwülste. Z. Krebsforsch. **33**, 594 (1930).

IRONS, H. S., JR.: Carcinoma twice in the same stomach. Gastroenterology **46**, 44 (1964).

MACDONALD, ELEANOR J.: Occurrence of multiple primary cancers in a population of 200,000. Acta Un. int. Cancr. **16**, 1702 (1960).

MOORE, J. R., and H. S. MORTON: Gastric carcinoma: A statistical review of 427 cases of carcinoma of the stomach from 1941 through 1950. Ann. Surg. **141**, 185 (1955).

OOTA, K., and M. TANAKA: Colliding carcinomas of the stomach (a consideration of histogenesis of single malignant tumor in general). Gann **43**, 210 (1952).

SCHELL, R. F., M. B. DOCKERTY, and M. W. COMFORT: Carcinoma of the stomach associated with pernicious anemia: A clinical and pathologic study. Surg. Gynec. Obstet. **98**, 710 (1954).

TEPERSON, J. A., L. S. ALTMAN, and B. KOGUT: Multiple heterogeneous carcinoma of the stomach. J. int. Coll. Surg. **17**, 374 (1952).

WALTERS, W., H. K. GRAY, and J. T. PRIESTLEY: Carcinoma and Other Malignant Lesions of the Stomach. Philadelphia: W. B. Saunders Company 1943, p. 351.

WARREN, S.: Multiple cancers of the human gastrointestinal tract. J. nat. Cancer Inst. **5**, 375 (1945).

—, and O. GATES: Multiple primary malignant tumors: A survey of the literature and a statistical study. Amer. J. Cancer. **16**, 1358 (1932).

7. Multicentric Carcinoid Tumors

The frequent multicentricity of carcinoids of the small intestine has long been documented. Indeed, in 1888 LUBARSCH established this tumor as a pathologic entity by describing two cases of carcinoid tumors of the ileum, in both of which the lesions were multicentric. In 1931 COOKE found that, including the cases which he reported, there were 115 cases of carcinoid tumors of the small intestine in the world literature. Of these, 37 (32.6%) were multicentric.

A total of 61 patients were found to have carcinoid tumors of the small intestine at the Mayo Clinic during the period of this study. Of this group, 12 patients (19.7%) had multicentric carcinoid tumors.

To enhance the information regarding this interesting neoplasm we have subsequently studied all cases of carcinoid tumor of the small intestine presenting at the Mayo Clinic before 1960 (MOERTEL and associates). Of a total of 209 patients reviewed, 29% had discrete multicentric neoplasms. Whereas some patients had only two lesions, the majority had three or more, and some had almost innumerable tumors studding a large portion of the small intestine. This incidence of 29% for grossly multicentric simultaneous lesions greatly exceeds that for any other malignant neoplasm. This feature of the carcinoid tumor assumes still greater interest in light of the previously mentioned high rate of association of cancers of different tissues of origin with the carcinoid tumor of the small intestine.

The degree of multicentricity of carcinoid tumors of the small intestine is not shared by carcinoids of other common sites of origin. Only 3 of 147 cases of carcinoid tumors of the rectum that we reviewed (CALDAROLA and associates) showed multiple lesions, and we have not observed multicentric carcinoids of the appendix. The coexistence of carcinoids of different sites of origin is likewise uncommon.

It is of interest that of 38 patients who had carcinoids first discovered at autopsy, only 4 (10.5 %) had multicentric lesions, whereas of 23 patients with carcinoids discovered at operation, 8 (34.8 %) had multicentric lesions. In the study by DOCKERTY and ASHBURN of metastasizing carcinoids, 5 of 13 patients (38.5 %) had multicentric lesions. It is not surprising that multicentricity seems to compound the hazard of metastasis and clinical symptoms nor that a single neoplasm of such low-grade malignancy is frequently discovered only as an incidental finding at autopsy.

With the exception of carcinoids, other multiple primary malignant neoplasms confined to the small intestine are exceedingly rare. None were present in our series, and in 1953 FELDMAN was able to collect only six cases from the literature.

References

CALDAROLA, V. T., R. J. JACKMAN, C. G. MOERTEL, and M. B. DOCKERTY: Carcinoid tumors of the rectum. Amer. J. Surg. 107, 844 (1964).

COOKE, H. H.: Carcinoid tumors of the small intestine. Arch. Surg. 22, 568 (1931).

DOCKERTY, M. B., and F. S. ASHBURN: Carcinoid tumors (so-called) of the ileum: Report of thirteen cases in which there was metastasis. Arch. Surg. 47, 221 (1943).

FELDMAN, MAURICE: Multiple primary carcinomas of small intestine: A review of the literature. Amer. J. dig. Dis. 20, 1 (1953).

LUBARSCH, OTTO: Über den primären Krebs des Ileum nebst Bemerkungen über das gleichzeitige Vorkommen von Krebs und Tuberculose. Virchows Arch. path. Anat. 111, 280 (1888).

MOERTEL, C. G., W. G. SAUER, M. B. DOCKERTY, and A. H. BAGGENSTOSS: Life history of the carcinoid tumor of the small intestine. Cancer (Philad.) 14, 901 (1961).

8. Multicentric Adenocarcinomas of the Colon and Rectum

Early reports of multiple cancers of the large bowel occurred in the later years of the nineteenth century. CZERNY has been recognized as reporting in 1880 the first case to appear in the world literature, whereas FENGER reported in 1888 the first case in the English literature. Subsequent case reports were scattered sparsely through the pages of recorded medicine. In 1930 BARGEN and RANKIN presented data on a series of 16 cases and warned the physician to be alert to the possible presence of a second lesion in a patient with known cancer of the colon. By 1944 SLAUGHTER was able to collect data on 116 cases from the literature; and he stated that, with the exception of the skin, the colon was the commonest site of multiple malignant neoplasms confined to the same organ. A review of the world literature to date reveals that the total of reported cases of multiple cancer of the colon has now swelled to greater than 1,000. The statistics presented in the large series reported are summarized in Table 22.

The variation in incidence from 0.6 to 6.4% stresses the need for a single series of cases extensive enough to give a more valid concept of the true frequency of

Table 22. *Incidence of Multiple Lesions in Reported Series of 100 or More Cases of Cancer of the Colon*

Reporting authors	Total cases of colonic cancer	Cases with multiple colonic cancer	Incidence %
THOMAS et al.	Not stated	132	3.0
POLK et al.	2,157	56	2.6
McGREGOR and BACON	1,788	94	5.3
MIDER et al.	1,129	40[1]	3.5
BRINDLEY and RICE	1,091	51	4.7
STENSTROM and FORD	1,000	48[1]	4.8
WILSON and TENNANT	950	44	4.6
ALBRECHT	848	12	1.4
TONDREAU	812	24	3.0
GARLOCK et al.	779	56[2]	7.2
SHALLOW et al.	750	44	5.9
GINZBURG and DREILING	700	25[2]	3.6
HIEL	635	5	0.8
SWINTON et al.	608	20	3.3
POSTLETHWAIT et al.	582	5	0.9
SPEAR and BRAINARD	568	10	1.8
WARREN	476	22	4.6
MacDONALD	446	20	4.5
RANKIN and JOHNSTON	438	3	0.7
BRODERS et al.	411	23	5.6
BERSON and BERGER	344	16	4.7
THORLAKSON	282	18	6.4
KIRSHBAUM and SHIVELY	173	2	1.2
BEHREND	158	1	0.6
PEABODY and SMITHWICK	100	7	7.0

[1] Included in situ carcinoma in adenomatous polyps.
[2] Interval lesions only.

multiple cancers of the colon. If this is indeed a common phenomenon, then the physician entrusted with the responsibility of diagnosis and treatment of these lesions should be provided with an abundance of clinical and pathologic knowledge. It may also be hoped that a study of patients with two or more malignant lesions of the colon may bring out in bolder relief etiologic and pathogenic features that are more obscure in patients with single lesions.

a) Selection of Cases

The pathologic findings were reviewed in all cases of adenocarcinoma of the colon or rectum proved at operation or from autopsy specimens seen at the Mayo Clinic during the 10-year period of this study. Cases were accepted as multiple cancers only if they met the following criteria:

Multiple Simultaneous Carcinomas

1. Each lesion must be of pathologically proved malignancy.

2. All lesions must be distinctly separated by normal bowel wall.

3. The possibility that one of the lesions represents a local extension or metastasis must be ruled out beyond any reasonable doubt.

Multiple Interval Carcinomas

1. Each lesion must be of pathologically proved malignancy.

2. The more recent lesion must be distinctly separated from the previous line of anastomosis.

3. The possibility that the more recent lesion represents a recurrence or metastasis must be ruled out beyond any reasonable doubt.

All lesions which were diagnosed within a 6-month period were arbitrarily classified as simultaneous, whereas all lesions discovered 6 months or longer after the initial lesion were classified as interval carcinomas.

The term "pathologically proved malignancy" is indeed controversial, particularly in regard to the low grade in situ malignant change found in adenomatous polyps. Opinions as to the true malignancy of such a lesion run the full gamut from complete denial to complete acceptance. A dogmatic and yet practical appraisal of this problem has been made by BUIE: "All polyps of the colon are cancers (carcinoma) or will become cancers if they are not destroyed or if the patient lives long enough. This extreme view is a safe one to hold, and there is much evidence, not always well controlled of course, to support it." It is not our intent to enter into this controversy; and in order to make the material presented here generally acceptable, only those cases will be included in which the lesions were felt to be unequivocally malignant by virtue of their invasiveness or high grade of malignancy. When pertinent, however, attention will be called to the association of low grade in situ malignant lesions with unequivocal carcinoma.

Microscopic examination of the intervening bowel wall was found to be an essential step in establishing the true multiplicity of closely neighboring lesions. In several cases in which the lesions were presumed to be multiple by gross examination, they were found by histologic examination to have extensive submucosal communications.

b) Results

A total of 6,012 patients were proved to have carcinomas of the colon or rectum during the 10-year period of this study. Of this group, a total of 261 patients were shown to have multiple lesions confirmed by the criteria listed in the previous section. Simultaneous lesions were found in 157 patients, interval lesions in 95, and simultaneous and interval lesions in 9. The rate of occurrence of multiple colonic cancer in this group is shown in Table 23.

If one considers low grade in situ carcinoma as representing a true malignant neoplasm, the overall occurrence of multiple lesions over the same 10-year period would be 985 cases (12.9 %) of a total of 7,664 cases of colonic cancer.

Multiple Simultaneous (Synchronous) Colonic Carcinomas. 1. Rate of Occurrence. — The incidence of multiple simultaneous colonic carcinoma is shown in Table 24. Of the 166 patients in this group, 132 had two lesions, 15 had three lesions, 12 had four lesions, and 4 had five lesions. In addition, three patients had diffusely scattered patches of high grade adenocarcinoma showing only early or no invasion. This pathologic pattern was confined to those patients who had associated chronic ulcerative colitis.

Table 23. *Multiple Colonic Carcinomas (Simultaneous and Interval): Rate of Occurrence According to Sex*

Patients	Total cases of colonic cancer	Cases of multiple colonic cancers	Rate of occurrence, %
Men	3,547	150	4.2
Women	2,465	111	4.5
Total	6,012	261	4.3

2. Age of occurrence. — The average age of diagnosis of multiple simultaneous carcinomas of the colon was 58.3 years in men and 54.8 years in women, or a combined average age of 56.7 years. For a 20-year period from 1926 through 1945, the average ages of patients seen at this clinic with malignant lesions of the large intestine were 57 years for men, 54 years for women, and just under 56 years for the entire series. On comparing these figures, it does not appear that there is a

Table 24. *Multiple Simultaneous Colonic Carcinomas: Rate of Occurrence According to Sex*

Patients	Total cases of colonic cancer	Multiple simultaneous colonic cancers	Rate of occurrence, %
Men	3,547	93	2.6
Women	2,465	73	3.0
Total	6,012	166	2.8

significant difference in the age of occurrence of single and multiple colonic carcinomas.

3. Location and Distribution of Lesions. — The percentage distribution of simultaneous lesions is shown in Figure 12. There can be no doubt about the marked tendency of simultaneous carcinomas to occur in the same region of the bowel. Twenty-eight per cent of the simultaneous lesions were confined to the same segment, and 68% to the same or an adjacent segment. This same pattern of distribution was even more striking in the cases of low grade in situ carcinoma in polyps associated with unequivocal carcinomas. These findings again support the concept that multiple colonic carcinomas do not occur as biologic accidents but rather are a multicentric form of the same basic malignant disease of the bowel. The fact that the largest portion of multiple lesions tend to be concentrated in the same region of bowel should not lull the surgeon into an attitude of complacency, however, since if only the same and adjacent segments are explored, about 32% of simultaneous lesions will be missed.

In Table 25 the overall distribution of simultaneous lesions is compared with the percentage distribution of more than 8,000 carcinomas of the large intestine as reported by MAYO. This comparison would seem to show that multiple lesions are proportionately less frequent in the rectum than in the more proximal colonic segments. This relation may be more apparent than real, however, since multiple

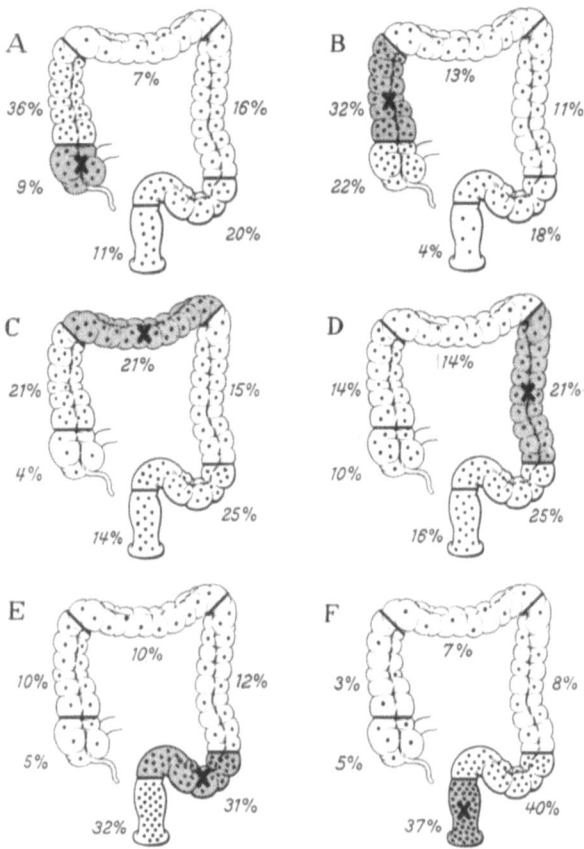

Fig. 12. Percentage distribution of carcinomas occurring simultaneously with carcinomas of (A) cecum, (B) ascending colon, (C) transverse colon, (D) descending colon, (E) sigmoid, and (F) rectum

lesions confined to the smaller rectal area would tend to fuse early in their develop-ment and thus not be acceptable to the criteria of this study.

Multiple Interval Colonic Carcinomas. — The possibility that, after a successful resection of one carcinoma of the colon, a patient may have a second entirely independent lesion is a contingency that no physician may ignore. There could be few errors more inexcusable than to assume falsely that such a second lesion was a metastasis or recurrence and to employ only palliative therapy.

1. Rate of Occurrence. — The existence of independent interval carcinomas of the colon was proved at this clinic in 104 patients during the 10-year period of this study. This figure is an obvious underestimate of the true incidence, since it does not include patients who may have had colonic carcinomas proved elsewhere prior or subsequent to the diagnosis of the lesion proved at this clinic, nor does it include patients who may have had second unproved lesions at the time of their subsequent

death. The percentage shown in Table 26, therefore, may be considered as only a lower limit to the true figure. Even if all interval colonic carcinomas could be included in a study such as this, the rate of occurrence as computed in Table 26

Table 25. *Regional Percentage Distribution of Multiple Simultaneous Colonic Carcinomas Compared With That of All Colonic Carcinomas*

Site of Lesion	Multiple simultaneous carcinomas	All carcinomas[1]
Cecum	10	5
Ascending colon and hepatic flexure	16	8
Transverse colon	10	6
Descending colon	12	7
Sigmoid	28	33
Rectum	24	41

[1] As adapted from MAYO.

would still be deceptively low, since it is calculated on the basis of all patients with colonic carcinomas rather than on the basis of patients who have survived their initial lesion.

Table 26. *Multiple Interval Colonic Carcinomas: Rate of Occurrence According to Sex*

Patients	Total colonic cancers	Multiple interval colonic cancers	Rate of occurrence, %
Men	3,547	63	1.8
Women	2,465	41	1.7
Total	6,012	104	1.7

2. Age of Occurrence. — The average age of occurrence and age range in interval colonic carcinomas are shown in Table 27. The average age of 53.8 years for the initial carcinoma is low when compared to 56 years, the average age of all patients

Table 27. *Multiple Interval Colonic Carcinomas: Age at Occurrence*

Patients	Lesion	Average age, yr	Age range, yr
Men	First	55.0	32—89
	Second	61.0	33—91
Women	First	52.0	22—80
	Second	57.5	25—84
Total average	First	53.8	22—89
	Second	59.6	25—91

who have colonic cancer. It would be unjustifiable to conclude from this, however, that patients who have malignant lesions of the colon at a younger age are more susceptible to the development of a second lesion. Patients of the older age groups have a higher incidence of other, unassociated causes of death, and are therefore less likely to live long enough to have a second lesion, even if they might have been so destined.

3. Interval Between Lesions. — The average interval in male patients with interval colonic carcinomas was 5.5 years with a range of 1 to 36 years; in female patients the average was 5.7 years with a range of 1 to 19 years. As can be seen in Fig. 13, the time when the physician should be most on guard against the occurrence of a second independent lesion is the time when he is most likely to be misled by the possibility of recurrence or metastasis. Twenty per cent of the second lesions occurred after only a 1-year interval, 45% within 3 years of the initial lesion, and 64% within 5 years.

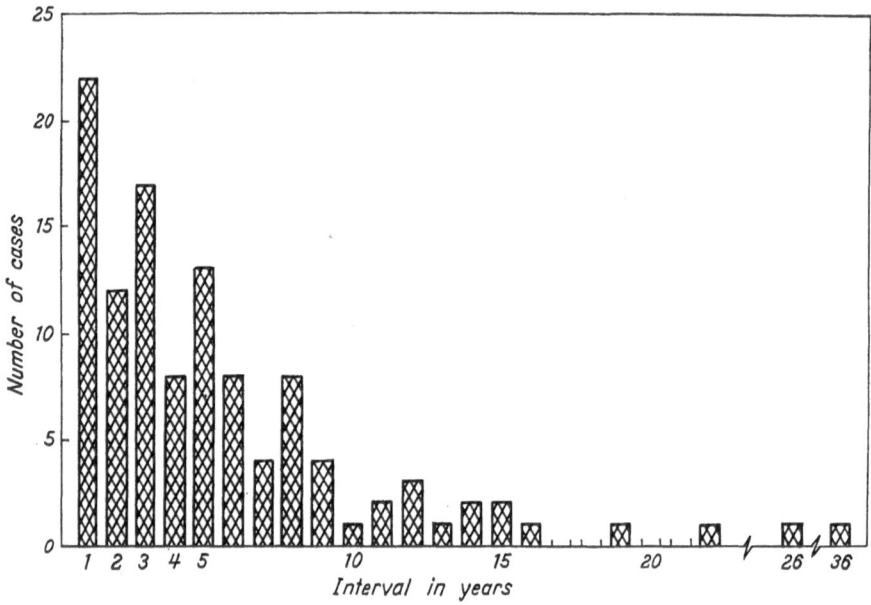

Fig. 13. Frequency distribution of cases of multiple interval colonic carcinomas by duration of interval between occurrence of the lesions

4. Location and Distribution of Lesions. — The distribution of initial lesions in patients with interval carcinomas of the colon or rectum, compared with that in the overall series, as adapted from Mayo, is shown in Table 28. The difference in representation of rectal carcinomas can probably be most easily explained by the fact that after surgical removal of a rectal carcinoma, the commonest sites of carcinoma of the large bowel have been removed.

The Association of Multiple Colonic Carcinomas With Other Colonic Lesions. — That multiple polyposis and chronic ulcerative colitis are etiologic or at least predisposing factors in the development of carcinoma of the colon, particularly in the younger age groups, seems well established. This relationship is brought out dramatically in patients with multiple colonic carcinomas, as is shown in Fig. 14.

1. Multiple Colonic Carcinomas and Multiple Polyposis. — During the 10-year period of this study, a total of 144 patients had either familial or apparently nonfamilial multiple polyposis, as proved by examination of surgical specimens at this clinic. Of this group, 13 patients (9%) had no evidence of malignant change, 60 (41%) had low grade in situ carcinomatous changes, 47 (33%) had single unequivocal carcinomas, and 24 (17%) had multiple carcinomas.

Malignant change and the development of multiple malignant lesions seem to be definitely associated with advancing age. The average age of patients showing no malignant change was 28 years; of patients showing only in situ carcinomatous changes, 36 years; of patients with single carcinoma, 43 years; and of patients with multiple carcinomas, 47 years.

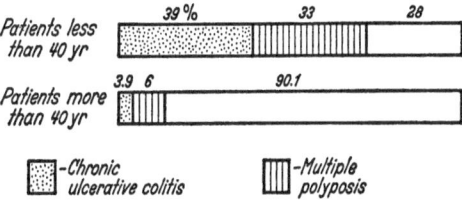

Fig. 14. The association of multiple colonic carcinomas with other colonic lesions

The urgent need for early diagnosis and radical treatment in these cases cannot be overemphasized. There seems to be no valid argument opposing the emphatic statement of Dixon: "Multiple carcinomas will develop in 100 per cent of neglected cases of polyposis of familial origin . . . ."

Table 28. *Regional Percentage Distribution of Multiple Interval Colonic Carcinomas, Initial Lesion, Compared With That of All Colonic Carcinomas*

Site of Lesion	Interval carcinomas, initial lesion	All carcinomas
Cecum	6	5
Ascending colon and hepatic flexure	13	8
Transverse colon	12	6
Descending colon	15	7
Sigmoid	36	33
Rectum	18	41

2. Multiple Colonic Carcinomas and Chronic Ulcerative Colitis. — The etiologic importance of chronic ulcerative colitis in the production of colonic carcinoma seems to be well supported by several studies in the recent literature. Probably the most impressive of these is the report by Bargen and associates of a follow-up study of 1,564 patients who had chronic ulcerative colitis. In 94 of these, colonic carcinoma developed at some later date. It was estimated that the frequency of colonic carcinoma in this group was 30 times that expected in the general population.

Of the 261 patients with multiple colonic carcinoma in the present study, a total of 24 (9%) had associated chronic ulcerative colitis. In general, these patients had lesions of a high grade of malignancy, and several had the distinctive pattern of multiple patches of high-grade adenocarcinoma replacing the mucosa and scattered over wide areas of the colon.

In studying 73 cases of adenocarcinoma of the colon associated with chronic ulcerative colitis seen at the Mayo Clinic, SHANDS and associates found multicentric carcinomas in 52.5% of 40 surgical specimens. This is approximately 20 times the incidence of multiple simultaneous carcinomas found in this study of all cases of

6*

colonic carcinoma. From this evidence, there can be little doubt that the coexistence of carcinoma of the colon and chronic ulcerative colitis is a strong indication for total colectomy.

The Association of Multiple Colonic Carcinomas With Other Malignant Disease. — Twenty-one patients (8 %) of the 261 patients in this study had additional primary malignant neoplasms entirely independent of their multiple colonic cancers. The location and frequency of occurrence of these lesions are listed in Table 29. The distribution of these neoplasms does not seem remarkable. These findings again illustrate the pitfalls in assuming any lesion to be a metastasis or a recurrence without pathologic confirmation.

Table 29. *Additional Primary Malignant Neoplasms Associated With Multiple Colonic Carcinomas*

Site of lesion	Cases	Site of lesion	Cases
Skin	3	Larynx	1
Breast	3	Jejunum	1
Bladder	3	Ileum (carcinoid)	1
Prostate	2	Hepatic duct	1
Ovary	2	Fibrosarcoma, subcutaneous	1
Stomach	1	Lymphosarcoma of vulva	1
Uterus	1		

Hereditary Influences in Multiple Colonic Carcinomas. — Although there is convincing evidence of hereditary factors in the genesis of malignant neoplasms in some experimental animals, there is little factual information to support the hypothesis of the influence of such factors on neoplasia in man. The difficulties encountered in attempting any large-scale, accurate, and well-controlled study in this regard are almost insurmountable.

It may be conjectured that hereditary influence in malignant disease may be magnified in patients who have multiple malignant neoplasms. The literature concerned with multiple primary cancers is liberally sprinkled with percentage figures on the family history of malignant disease, as given by the patients included in the particular series reported. It is obviously impossible to draw any conclusions from any single figure for family incidence, since this is in large part determined by the diligence of the examining physician and the intelligence of the patients.

The study to follow suffers from all the limitations and inaccuracies of any study based on secondhand information obtained in medical histories. It is hoped that many of these limitations may be negated by the use of a large group of patients and by the use of control groups. Here again, however, even the most carefully chosen control groups must always be subject to question when one is dealing with such a nebulous entity as hereditary influence in malignant disease.

The family histories obtained in the admission interviews of more than 1,000 patients were studied, and data regarding more than 3,000 family members were recorded. Only information regarding the immediate family (parents, siblings, and children) was used. Data regarding a family member were recorded only if the patient had stated the present age or the age at death of the family member. A family member was recorded as having malignant disease only if there was an unequivocal statement confirming the presence of cancer; vague terms such as "tumor" were not accepted. The patients and their corresponding family members were then gathered into three groups:

1. Group I (195 Patients). — Patients who had unequivocal multiple carcinomas of the colon or rectum which had been proved at the Mayo Clinic from January 1, 1944, through December 31, 1953. (Patients who had multiple polyposis were not included in this study.)

2. Group II (414 Patients). — Patients who had single carcinoma of the colon or rectum which had been proved at this clinic from January 1, 1944, through December 31, 1953. The sex ratio, average age at the time of diagnosis, and age distribution are the same as in group I. The grade of malignancy and location of lesions are represented in the same proportion as in group I.

3. Group III (414 Patients). — Patients seen at this clinic from January 1, 1944, through December 31, 1953, who gave no history of previous malignant disease and who on examination showed no evidence of malignant disease. The sex ratio, average age, and age distribution are the same as in groups I and II.

There was no significant difference in the overall incidence of malignant disease in these three groups. However, when this incidence was plotted against the reported age of these family members, a definite trend seemed to be established (Fig. 15). Malignant disease seemed to occur at an earlier age in relatives of patients with colonic carcinoma than in relatives of patients without malignant disease. This tendency, while only slight in group II, seems quite definite in group I.

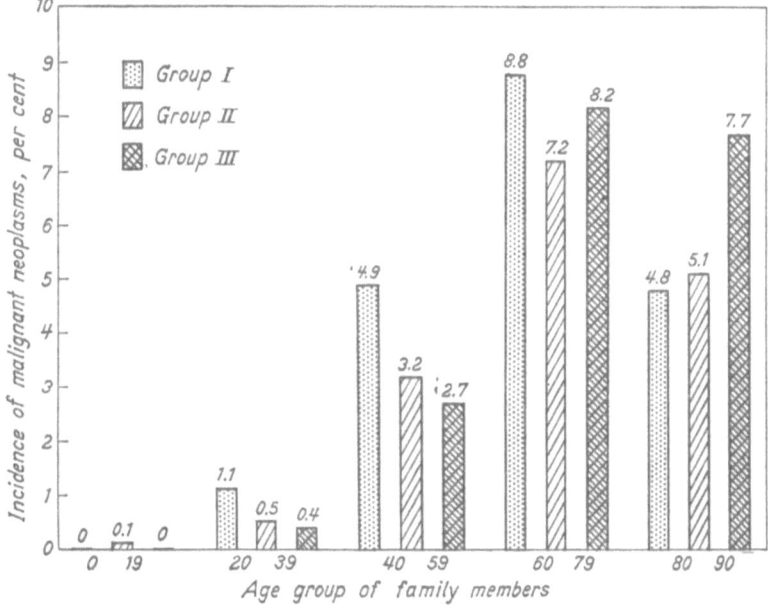

Fig. 15. Comparative familial incidence of malignant neoplasms by age of family members (see text)

When the specific types of malignant disease stated for the family members are tabulated, a still more striking difference in the three groups is manifested (Fig. 16).

If one may draw a general conclusion from this limited study, it would be that the hereditary influence in colonic carcinoma is evidenced by an earlier age of development of malignant disease in members of families of patients who have

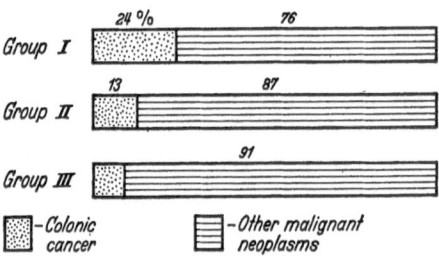

Fig. 16. Relative frequency of colonic cancer among family members with malignant neoplasms (see text)

malignant disease of the colon, and that this hereditary influence is in some measure specific for colonic carcinoma. It is interesting that this pattern is analogous to that seen in a more exaggerated form in families of patients who have multiple polyposis. Indeed, it may be that the familial pattern described here applies more correctly to the formation of the premalignant adenomatous polyp rather than directly to the formation of colonic carcinoma per se.

c) Comment

This study, as well as others, has amply demonstrated that in a significant proportion of cases colonic carcinoma is multicentric. This fact, however, should not be tucked away in the pages of pathology texts and disregarded in the practical management of patients who have carcinoma of the large bowel. Any physician who accepts the responsibility of treating this disease must also accept the responsibility of maintaining a constant vigil to discover and promptly treat any simultaneous or interval lesions. The rate of occurrence of at least 1.7% of interval carcinomas presented in this study cannot be ignored. That this may represent only a small fraction of the true rate of occurrence of interval lesions has been suggested by the study of Long and associates. In a study of 31 lesions previously diagnosed as recurrences occurring at the site of anastomosis, they found that 9 lesions had a transition zone of anaplastic cells between the main carcinoma and the normal bowel mucosa. They concluded that this transition zone established these lesions as new and independent growths. Schweiger and Bargen have speculated as to what proportion of poor results after operation for colonic cancer are attributable to synchronous or metachronous lesions, unsuspected and therefore undiscovered.

To ensure early and adequate treatment of second lesions in patients with known colonic carcinoma, the following program is suggested as the minimal requirements for management of all patients who have carcinoma of the large bowel:

1. The entire colon and rectum must be carefully examined at the time of treatment of the initial lesion. This examination should include direct visualization of as much of the mucosa as is practicable.

2. Multiple polyposis and carcinoma complicating chronic ulcerative colitis should be positive indications for total colectomy.

3. All polyps should be promptly treated by resection or fulguration as soon as possible after their discovery.

4. The physician must assume the responsibility for impressing the patient with the necessity for frequent and regular follow-up examinations. These examinations must be done at no longer than 1-year intervals for at least 5 years after treatment of the initial lesion and preferably at yearly intervals thereafter.

5. A minimal follow-up examination must include a proctoscopic examination as well as a careful roentgenologic examination of the colon.

Summary

The literature concerning multiple colonic carcinomas has been reviewed.

Data have been presented on 261 cases in which multiple carcinomas of the colon were seen at the Mayo Clinic from January 1, 1944, through December 31, 1953. This represents a known rate of occurrence of 4.3 %.

A marked tendency to multiplicity has been observed in carcinoma of the colon associated with multiple polyposis or with chronic ulcerative colitis.

Some evidence has been obtained of hereditary factors in predisposition to malignant disease of the colon.

When the diagnosis of a malignant lesion of the colon or rectum has been made, the entire large bowel must be considered a potential source of malignant disease. An integral part of the management of carcinoma of the large bowel must be constant vigilance to ensure early diagnosis and adequate treatment of both simultaneous and interval lesions.

References

ALBRECHT, P.: Über die Multiplizität primärer maligner Geschwülste. Oncologia (Basel) 5, 12 (1952).

BARGEN, J. A., and F. W. RANKIN: Multiple carcinomata of the large intestine. Ann. Surg. 91, 583 (1930).

—, W. G. SAUER, W. P. SLOAN, and R. P. GAGE: The development of cancer in chronic ulcerative colitis. Gastroenterology 26, 32 (1954).

BEHREND, M.: Carcinoma of colon: Treatment depending on location of lesions. Surg. Gynec. Obstet. 65, 505 (1937).

BERSON, H. L., and L. BERGER: Multiple carcinomas of the large intestine. Surg. Gynec. Obstet. 80, 75 (1945).

BRINDLEY, G. V., and J. S. RICE, JR.: Multiple primary malignancies of the large intestine. Surg. Clin. N. Amer. 32, 1499 (1952).

BRODERS, A. C., C. PHILLIPS, and J. C. STINSON: Neoplasms of the large bowel. Surg. Clin. N. Amer. 32, 1511 (1952).

BUIE, L. A.: Polypoid disease of the colon. Postgrad. Med. 5, 177 (1949).

CZERNY: II. Aus der Heidelberger chirurgischen Klinik: Nachtrag zur Darmresection. Berl. klin. Wschr. 17, 683 (1880).

DIXON, C. F.: Malignant lesions of the colon: Preoperative and postoperative management with comment on prognosis. Surg. Clin. N. Amer. 31, 1013 (1951).

FENGER, C.: Double carcinoma of the colon. J. Amer. med. Ass. 11, 606 (1888).

GARLOCK, J. H., BERNARD LERMAN, S. H. KLEIN, A. S. LYONS, and P. A. KIRSCHNER: Twenty-five years' experience with surgical therapy of cancer of the colon and rectum: An analysis of 1,887 cases. Dis. Colon Rect. 5, 247 (1962).

GINZBURG, L., and D. A. DREILING: Successive independent (metachronous) carcinomas of the colon. Ann. Surg. 143, 117 (1956).

HIEL, M.: Cancers primitifs multiples rectocoliques et association d'une tumeur gastrique à une tumeur rectocolique. Acta chir. belg. 52, 777 (1953).

KIRSHBAUM, J. D., and F. L. SHIVELY, JR.: Multiple primary malignant tumors. J. Lab. clin. Med. 24, 283 (1938).

LONG, J. W., C. W. MAYO, M. B. DOCKERTY, and E. S. JUDD, JR.: Recurrent versus new and independent carcinomas of the colon and rectum. Proc. Mayo Clin. 25, 169 (1950).

MACDONALD, ELEANOR J.: Occurrence of multiple primary cancers in a population of 200,000. Acta Un. int. Cancr. 16, 1702 (1960).

MAYO, C. W.: Surgery of the colon: Selection of patients and operations for malignant lesions. Postgrad. Med. 5, 394 (1949).

McGREGOR, R. A., and H. E. BACON: Multiple cancers in colon surgery: Report of 162 cases. Surgery 44, 828 (1958).

MIDER, G. B., J. A. SCHILLING, J. C. DONOVAN, and E. S. RENDALL: Multiple cancer: A study of other cancers arising in patients with primary malignant neoplasms of the stomach, uterus, breast, large intestine, or hematopoietic system. Cancer (Philad.) 5, 1104 (1952).

PEABODY, C. N., and R. H. SMITHWICK: Practical implications of multiple tumors of the colon and rectum. New Engl. J. Med. 264, 853 (1961).

POLK, H. C., JR., J. S. SPRATT, JR., and H. R. BUTCHER, JR.: Frequency of multiple primary malignant neoplasms associated with colorectal carcinoma. Amer. J. Surg. 109, 71 (1965).

POSTLETHWAIT, R. W., J. E. ADAMSON, and DERYL HART: Carcinoma of the colon and rectum. Surg. Gynec. Obstet. 106, 257 (1958).

RANKIN, F. W., and C. C. JOHNSTON: II. Multiple malignant lesions of the large bowel. Int. Clin. 4. 2, 246 (1941).

SCHWEIGER, L. R., and J. A. BARGEN: Multiple primary malignant lesions of the large bowel. Arch. intern. Med. 66, 1331 (1940).

SHALLOW, T. A., F. B. WAGNER, JR., and R. E. COLCHER: Clinical evaluation of 750 patients with colon cancer: Diagnostic survey and follow-up covering a fifteen-year period. Ann. Surg. 142, 164 (1955).

SHANDS, W. C., M. B. DOCKERTY, and J. A. BARGEN: Adenocarcinoma of the large intestine associated with chronic ulcerative colitis: Clinical and pathologic features of 73 cases. Surg. Gynec. Obstet. 94, 302 (1952).

SLAUGHTER, D. P.: The multiplicity of origin of malignant tumors: Collective review. Int. Abstr. Surg. 79, 89 (1944).

SPEAR, H. C., and S. C. BRAINARD: Cancer of the large bowel — an analysis of 580 lesions. Ann. Surg. 134, 934 (1951).

STENSTROM, J. D., and H. S. FORD: Carcinoma of the colon: Analysis of 1,000 cases with particular reference to polyps and multiple carcinoma. Amer. J. Surg. 88, 200 (1954).

SWINTON, N. W., ENRIQUE MOSZKOWSKI, and J. C. SNOW: Cancer of the colon and rectum: A statistical study of 608 patients. Surg. Clin. N. Amer. 39, 745 (1959).

THOMAS, J. F., M. B. DOCKERTY, and J. M. WAUGH: Multiple primary carcinomas of the large intestine. Cancer (Philad.) 1, 564 (1948).

THORLAKSON, P. H. T.: The incidence of multiple malignant growths of the large bowel. Manitoba med. Rev. 32, 158 (1952).

TONDREAU, R. L.: Multiple primary carcinomas of the large intestine. Amer. J. Roentgen. 71, 794 (1954).

WARREN, S.: Multiple cancers of the human gastrointestinal tract. J. nat. Cancer Inst. 5, 375 (1945).

WILSON, J. S., and ROBERT TENNANT: Carcinoma of the colon: A 10-year study. Cancer (Philad.) 11, 278 (1958).

9. Multicentric Epitheliomas of the Urinary Tract

The striking frequency of multiple papillary epitheliomas of the urinary tract has been recognized for many years. In 1934 the Committee on Carcinoma Registry reported that of 902 cases of bladder cancer reported to the tumor registry of the American Urological Association, 259 cases (29%) presented with multiple lesions.

A more recent study in 1955 by MELICOW reported that of 270 patients with vesical tumors treated by fulguration, 65 had multiple lesions at the time of the initial examination, an incidence of 24%. This tendency to multiplicity of tumors seems to apply equally to the remainder of the urinary tract. OPPENHEIMER and LEAR stated that 33% of the renal papillary tumors also are found to be associated with papillary lesions on cystoscopic examination. In 48 (36%) of 133 cases of tumor of the renal pelvis studied, KAPLAN and associates found multiple lesions of the urinary tract.

Although theories of epithelial extension and lymphatic metastasis have been offered to explain this phenomenon, the predominant line of controversy in recent literature has been drawn between those favoring implantation of exfoliated tumor cells from a single primary lesion and those favoring multicentric origin of the papillary neoplasms. Many feel that implantation can and probably does occur in areas of the bladder that have beeen traumatized and denuded of mucosa during fulguration of a neoplasm. MCDONALD and THORSON demonstrated the transplantability of vesical tumors in the dog if the cells are allowed to incubate in a surgically produced stagnant pouch. It is still unproved, however, whether such implantation can take place on intact urinary epithelium that has not been subjected to prior surgical manipulation in the presence of a constant urinary flow.

As evidence against implantation, BRODERS has shown that in the so-called implants there is continuity between the tumor and the basal cells of the mucosa which seems to indicate that the tumors originated in the basal layer and were not implanted on the surface of the epithelium. Other studies of this problem, such as those of WILLIS, EWING, MELICOW (1944), and MCDONALD and PRIESTLEY, have strengthened the concept that multicentric origin is the most acceptable explantation for the occurrence of multiple tumors of the urinary epithelium.

a) Multicentric Tumors of the Bladder

In the present study, 36 cases of multiple epitheliomas of the bladder were found. This is in no way representative of the true frequency of multiple tumors of the bladder seen at this clinic during the period of study. Our criteria stated that a discrete specimen from each lesion must be obtained and examined if the case was to be included in the group. In most cases of this type, the treatment is fulguration, and pathologic examination is made on a single specimen or on an aggregate of all tissue removed. These specimens were not acceptable as giving evidence of multiple tumors according to the criteria of this study. Cases included are largely those in which partial or total cystectomy permitted examination of each lesion as well as the intervening bladder wall.

In order to obtain a more accurate estimation of the frequency of multiplicity of bladder tumors, we studied 112 consecutive cases of proved cancer of the bladder initially diagnosed at the Mayo Clinic during a 1-year period. Patients were not included if they had had previously treated cancer of the bladder. Of these 112 patients, 21 (19%) were found to have multiple vesical tumors at the time of the initial cystoscopic examination at this clinic.

MELICOW, as well as the Committee on Carcinoma Registry, demonstrated that the presence of multicentricity when the patient is initially treated has a great influence on the subsequent recurrence rate of vesical tumors. Sixty-six of our

112 patients were reexamined at this clinic at intervals of 1 or more years after treatment of their initial malignant neoplasm or neoplasms. Eighteen of the 44 patients who initially had had single lesions (41 %) had proved recurrences, and 10 of the 12 who initially had had multiple lesions (83 %) had proved recurrences.

The number of so-called recurrences of bladder cancers that are in fact new and independent lesions is open to conjecture. EWING stated that it is probable that the recurrence usually represents a development of a new tumor from preexisting lesions, not a recrudescence or implantation of the old growth.

b) Multicentric Lesions Associated with Neoplasms of the Renal Pelvis [1]

A total of 95 patients with pathologically proved carcinomas of the renal pelvis were seen at this clinic during the 10-year period covered by this study. Seven of these patients (7.4 %) had multiple discrete epitheliomas confined to the same renal pelvis. Thirty-three (35 %) had associated lesions in the lower part of the urinary tract (ureter, bladder, or urethra). In 14 of these latter cases the lesion of the renal pelvis and lower part of the urinary tract were diagnosed simultaneously. In 10 patients the renal pelvic lesion preceded the lesion lower in the urinary tract by periods of 1 to 3 years. Results of cystoscopic examination on all of these patients were negative at the time of diagnosis of the epithelioma of the kidney. In eight patients lesions of the bladder preceded the lesion of the renal pelvis by 2 to 6 years; all of these had had negative excretory urograms at the time of treatment of the bladder lesion. These last eight cases would be difficult to explain by any theory except that the lesions arose as a multicentric response to a common carcinogenic influence.

All of the statistics given herein as well as those in the literature support the conclusion of FERRIS and associates that "persistent and frequent surveys of the urinary tract are imperative in cases in which a papillary neoplasm has been found ... ."

References

BRODERS, A. C.: Discussion. Proc. Mayo Clin. **13**, 499 (1938).

COMMITTEE ON CARCINOMA REGISTRY: Cancer of the bladder: A study based on 902 epithelial tumors of the bladder in the carcinoma registry of the American Urological Association. J. Urol. (Baltimore) **31**, 423 (1934).

EWING, JAMES: Neoplastic Diseases, Ed. 3. Philadelphia: W. B. Saunders Company 1934, pp. 909—910.

FERRIS, D. O., J. H. KAPLAN, and G. J. THOMPSON: Papillary epitheliomas in each ureter and in the bladder. J. Urol. (Baltimore) **62**, 448 (1949).

KAPLAN, J. H., J. R. McDONALD, and G. J. THOMPSON: Multicentric origin of papillary tumors of the urinary tract. J. Urol. (Baltimore) **66**, 792 (1951).

McDONALD, D. F., and THEODORE THORSON: Clinical implications of transplantability of induced bladder tumors to intact transitional epithelium of dogs. J. Urol. (Baltimore) **75**, 690 (1956).

McDONALD, J. R., and J. T. PRIESTLEY: Carcinoma of the renal pelvis: Histopathologic study of seventy-five cases with special reference to prognosis. J. Urol. (Baltimore) **51**, 245 (1944).

---

[1] Cases encountered prior to 1947 have been reported previously by KAPLAN and co-workers.

MELICOW, M. M.: Classification of renal neoplasms: A clinical and pathological study based on 199 cases. J. Urol. (Baltimore) 51, 333 (1944).
— Tumors of the urinary bladder: A clinicopathological analysis of over 2500 specimens and biopsies. J. Urol. (Baltimore) 74, 498 (1955).
OPPENHEIMER, G. D., and HAROLD LEAR: Papillary carcinoma of the ureter and bladder thirteen years post-nephrectomy for papillary carcinoma of the kidney. J. Mt Sinai Hosp. 17, 671 (1951).
WILLIS, R. A.: Pathology of Tumours. St. Louis: C. V. Mosby Company 1948, p. 470.

10. Multicentric Carcinomas of the Cervix, Vagina, Vulva, and Anus

The vulva, vagina, anus, and portio vaginalis of the cervix share a contiguous surface of squamous epithelium derived from the same embryologic anlage. Thus, on the basis of exposure to a common carcinogenic influence or of a common intrinsic susceptibility to malignant change, multicentric carcinomas may be anticipated in these areas.

This predicted tendency to multicentricity was found to be especially marked for squamous cell carcinomas of the vulva and vagina. From the total of 137 patients with carcinoma of the vulva or vagina proved at the Mayo Clinic during the 10-year period of this study, eight (5.8%) had two or more discrete lesions confined to the vulva and vagina. In addition, nine patients had associated squamous cell carcinomas of the cervix, and one patient had a squamous cell carcinoma of the anus. The overall occurrence rate of multicentric lesions among women with carcinomas of the vulva and vagina was 16 (11.7%) of 137 patients. An even more striking incidence of multicentricity was observed by GREEN and associates. By gross and histologic studies they demonstrated multicentric foci of origin in 47 (19.7%) of 238 patients with epidermoid carcinoma of the vulva.

A similar but less pronounced tendency to involvement of these contiguous epithelial surfaces was observed in patients with squamous cell carcinomas of the cervix. Of 823 women with carcinoma of the cervix, a total of nine (1.1%) had discrete squamous cell carcinomas of the vulva or vagina. These 9 made up 15.5% of the 58 women in this series with carcinoma of the cervix who had an additional primary cancer, whereas less than 1% of all women with malignant disease seen at the Mayo Clinic during the period of this study had carcinomas of the vulva and vagina.

Reference

GREEN, T. H., JR., HOWARD ULFELDER, and J. V. MEIGS: Epidermoid carcinoma of the vulva: An analysis of 238 cases. Part I. Etiology and diagnosis. Part II. Therapy and end results. Amer. J. Obstet. Gynec. 75, 834 (1958).

11. Bilateral Carcinomas of the Breast

Bilateral mammary carcinoma has been the subject of much interest and controversy in medical literature for several decades. Probably the earliest reported observation of this phenomenon was recorded by NISBET in 1800. The credibility of his report, however, is the subject of some doubt, since he claimed to have cured the lesions in both breasts by the local application of an undisclosed medicament.

Much of the early literature is clouded by the lack of a clear distinction between cancerous lesions in the second breast which are in all likelihood separate and independent neoplasms and those lesions representing metastasis or local extension from a single malignant focus. The first clear-cut presentation of this problem was made by KILGORE in 1921. He discussed 37 cases of bilateral involvement among a total of 1,100 cases of cancer of the breast. He estimated that cancer is three to four times more likely to develop in the one remaining breast of the patient who has survived removal of cancer in a single breast than in either breast of a normal woman of the same age. In a similar analysis in 1952 MIDER and associates estimated the incidence of cancer in the second breast to be three and a half times that expected by chance alone. Reports such as these have led several authors to consider prophylactic simple mastectomy of the remaining breast as a means of increasing the overall effectiveness of surgical treatment of mammary cancer.

Practical justification for such an innovation would depend largely on the true frequency of occurrence of independent nonsynchronous cancer in the second breast. In 1955 CARROLL and SHIELDS reviewed the literature and found 1,059 cases of carcinoma in the second breast reported in 14 different series. The average incidence of independent cancer in the second breast according to these reports was 3.3 %. Such a figure is of limited value, however, because of the varied criteria used in the respective reports. Probably the most significant single series is that of HARRINGTON, who reported that cancer had developed in the remaining breast in 212 of 6,149 cases of mammary cancer encountered at the Mayo Clinic from 1910 to 1940, a rate of occurrence of 3.4 %.

The primary purposes of this presentation are (1) to establish simple and practical criteria for the diagnosis of independent cancer in the second breast in the hope that their use may standardize subsequent literature on this subject, and (2) to present the study of a large series of patients with cancer in the second breast confirmed by these criteria.

a) Criteria for the Diagnosis of Independent Cancer in the Second Breast

It is obvious that with our present knowledge of cancer biology no criteria can be established to distinguish with absolute certainty a primary carcinoma in the second breast from a metastatic lesion, except possibly in special circumstances such as bilateral comedocarcinomas. Criteria must be chosen which are neither so liberal that results of a study are questionable nor so rigid that the practical clinical value of the study is lost. Criteria also must be sufficiently objective to allow comparison of studies of various investigators. With these factors in mind, the following criteria were established for choosing the cases of unsimultaneous (nonsynchronous) cancer in the second breast to be reported herein:

1. Each lesion must be proved to be of unequivocal malignancy by pathologic examination.

2. The first lesion must have been removed by mastectomy with reasonable hope of cure at least 6 months prior to the diagnosis of the second lesion.

3. At the time of diagnosis of the most recent lesion, there must not be any evidence of local recurrence of the initial lesion or of distant metastasis.

The term "reasonable hope of cure" is intended to eliminate only those carcinomas which are far advanced or of inflammatory type so that mastectomy is performed largely for palliative purposes. The 6-month interval was chosen arbitrarily in an attempt to eliminate small lesions in the second breast which may have been present but undiagnosed at the time of the initial operation. In essence, the existence of carcinoma in the second breast must be proved and a second mastectomy with reasonable hope of long-term survival must be justified.

GUISS suggested the following condition as a necessary criterion: "The clinical course of the patient after the second radical mastectomy must be compatible with that of a primary lesion." At the Mayo Clinic, patients have been seen in whom extensive metastasis has developed rapidly and has led to death within a few months after radical mastectomy for carcinoma in a single breast. On the other hand, one patient has been seen in whom local recurrence developed in the scar 31 years after mastectomy, and another who first showed metastasis in a regional lymph node 29 years after mastectomy. With such wide variations, the definition of a course "compatible with a primary lesion" must be highly subjective at best.

The criteria established for recognition of cases of simultaneous (synchronous) cancer in the second breast to be reported herein are as follows:

1. Each lesion must be proved by pathologic examination to be of unequivocal malignancy.

2. Cases are acceptable only if there is no evidence of distant metastasis and minimal or no metastasis to regional lymph nodes.

3. Cases in which one or both lesions are located in the inner hemispheres are acceptable only if there is a distinct difference in microscopic morphologiy of the two lesions, or if intraductile cancer can be demonstrated in each breast.

Since these cases do not have the factor of an interval of time during which the patient can be demonstrated to be free of metastasis, the criteria for independent bilateral simultaneous breast cancers must be more rigid. This is demonstrated by the fact that by including all cases with mastectomy for bilateral simultaneous breast cancers, HARRINGTON could report a 5-year survival rate of only 28.8 % of 52 cases.

Unless the malignant disease is widespread, it would be difficult to conceive of a lesion in the outer quadrant of one breast giving rise to an isolated metastatic lesion in an outer quadrant of the opposite breast. Such is not the case, however, when malignant disease involves the inner quadrants, since lymphatic pathways may cross the sternum from these regions.

b) Observations

Of 2,945 patients who underwent mastectomy for cancer of the breast at this clinic from January 1, 1944, to January 1, 1954, a total of 118 patients were proved to have primary cancers in both breasts according to the established criteria. This represents an overall rate of occurrence of 4.0 %.

c) Unsimultaneous (Nonsynchronous) Cancer in the Second Breast

Rate of Occurrence (Table 30). — A total of 110 patients were found to have had unsimultaneous cancers in the second breast during the 10-year period of study. This group included 109 women and 1 man. The known rate of occurrence of these cancers during the 10-year period was 3.7 % (109 of 2,933 women or 3.7 %; 1 of

12 men or 8.3%). This slight increase over the rate reported by HARRINGTON probably reflects the improved survival rate for patients treated for cancer of the breast since the earlier years of this century.

Table 30. *Unsimultaneous Cancer of the Second Breast: Rate of Occurrence as Observed at the Mayo Clinic*

	Total patients with cancer of the breast	Patients with cancer in the second breast	Rate of occurrence, %
Study of HARRINGTON, 1910 to 1940	6,361	212	3.3
Present study, 1944 to 1954	2,945	110	3.7

It must be emphasized that this percentage (3.7%) represents only the *known rate of occurrence* of unsimultaneous cancer of the breast. Patients who may have had carcinoma of the second breast diagnosed and treated elsewhere, either prior or subsequent to cancer of the breast proved here, were not included in this study unless the surgical specimen or a portion thereof was submitted to this clinic for pathologic examination. Neither were patients included who may have had a second independent cancerous lesion in the breast but who also had evidence of distant metastasis at the time the second lesion was diagnosed at this clinic.

It must be emphasized also that 3.7% represents the known occurrence of bilateral unsimultaneous lesions among *all* patients who had undergone mastectomy for cancer of the breast. This figure is deceptively low since many of the patients having cancer of one breast died as a result of their initial lesion. A more realistic figure would be the rate of occurrence among patients who survived their initial mammary cancer. This would be impossible to obtain with statistical validity in this study. HARRINGTON has estimated the true incidence of bilateral unsimultaneous cancer of the breast to be between 6 and 8%, which would not seem to be an unreasonable estimate.

Age at Occurrence. — The average age of the patient at the time of occurrence of the initial cancerous lesion in the breast was 50.3 years; ages ranged from 29 to 75 years. This is not significantly different from the average age of 51.3 years reported by HARRINGTON for 6,195 women with cancer of one breast. The probability of cancer in the second breast, therefore, cannot be predicted by the patient's age when the first mammary cancer develops. The averge age at diagnosis of cancer in the second breast was 56.6 years, and ages ranged from 31 to 83 years.

Interval Between Lesions. — The average interval between diagnosis of cancer in the first and in the second breast was 6.3 years with a range of 7 months to 22 years. As is shown graphically in Figure 17, the frequency of occurrence of unsimultaneous cancers seems to vary in an inverse manner with the time that has elapsed after the diagnosis of the initial lesion: 23% of the lesions had occurred after a 1-year interval (± 6 months), 45% after a 3-year interval, and 57% after a 5-year interval. The remaining 43% developed after intervals ranging from 6 to 22 years.

Prognosis. — Of the 110 patients with nonsynchronous cancer of the breast, 84 had had a second mastectomy 5 or more years prior to the initial writing of this report and thus could potentially be traced for 5 years after the treatment of their second cancer. Adequate follow-up information was obtained on all 84 patients. The survival rate for this group (56.0%) is presented in Table 31 as is the rate for a group of patients having cancer in one breast only (60.3%). On comparison of

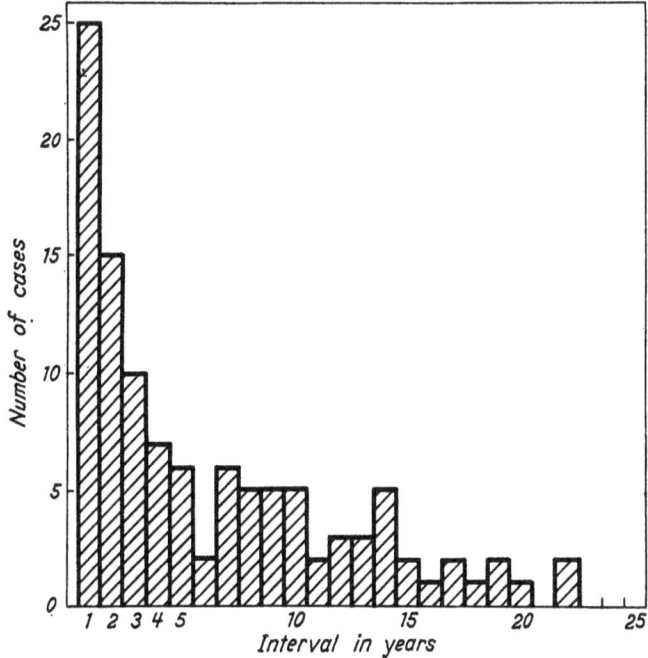

Fig. 17. Occurrence of independent cancer in the second breast, showing intervals between diagnosis of first and second/lesions in 110 cases

these survival rates it would appear that from an overall prognostic standpoint there is little difference in the course of patients after cancer develops in one breast only and that of patients after a nonsynchronous cancer develops in the second breast.

Table 31. *Comparison of Survival Rates After Mastectomy for Primary Cancer in One Breast and After Mastectomy for Independent Unsimultaneous Cancer in the Second Breast*

	Patients traced	Patients surviving 5 years or more	
		Number	%
Primary cancer in one breast: study of Pierce and associates, 1947 and 1948	634	382	60.3
Unsimultaneous cancer in second breast: present study, 1944 to 1951	84	47	56.0

It also would seem to be strong evidence that nonsynchronous cancer in the second breast chosen by the criteria listed herein does indeed represent an independent lesion.

d) Simultaneous (Synchronous) Cancer in the Second Breast

In only eight cases could the lesions be confirmed by the aforementioned criteria as independent simultaneous cancer in the second breast. All patients were women and their ages ranged from 44 to 73 years with an average age of 55.4 years. These

8 patients represent an incidence of 0.27 % among the total of 2,945 patients who had had mastectomy for cancer during the 10-year period of this study.

The clinical and pathologic findings in these eight cases are presented briefly:

Case 1. — A 65-year-old woman had an adenocarcinoma, grade 3, in the upper outer quadrant of the left breast without nodal involvement. A small cell adenocarcinoma, grade 4, was present in the upper outer quadrant of the right breast without nodal involvement. Evidence of distant metastasis was not found. The patient was alive and well 8 years after bilateral radical mastectomy.

Case 2. — A 69-year-old woman was found to have an adenocarcinoma, grade 4, in the extreme upper outer quadrant of the left breast without nodal involvement. In the right breast an adenocarcinoma, grade 4, was located in the upper outer quadrant without nodal involvement. An intraductile component was noted in the lesions of both breasts; distant metastasis was not evident. The patient died, presumably from metastasis, 4 years after bilateral radical mastectomy.

Case 3. — Examination of a woman 44 years of age showed an adenocarcinoma, grade 4, in the upper outer quadrant of the left breast with involvement of one axillary node. The right breast contained an adenocarcinoma, grade 4, in the upper quadrant; no nodes were involved. The lesions in both breasts contained intraductile components. Evidence of distant metastasis could not be found. The patient was alive and well 4½ years after bilateral radical mastectomy.

Case 4. — The left breast of a 47-year-old woman contained a scirrhous adenocarcinoma, grade 4, in the upper outer quadrant with early involvement of two axillary nodes. A comedoadenocarcinoma, grade 3, had developed in the upper outer quadrant of the right breast without nodal involvement. An intraductile component was contained in both lesions. Distant metastasis was not found. The patient underwent bilateral radical mastectomy and was alive and well 6 years later.

Case 5. — A scirrhous adenocarcinoma, grade 3, was located in the upper outer quadrant of the left breast of a 47-year-old woman. Early involvement of two axillary nodes was noted. The right breast contained a comedoadenocarcinoma, grade 3, in the upper outer quadrant, and two axillary nodes of this breast also showed evidence of early involvement. Intraductile components were present in the lesions of both breasts. Evidence of distant metastasis could not be found. The patient died of acute myocardial infarction 1 year after bilateral radical mastectomy.

Case 6. — Comedoadenocarcinomas, grade 3, were located in both breasts of a 44-year-old woman. In the left breast the lesion was situated directly under the nipple. In the right breast it was in the upper outer quadrant. Nodal involvement was not present in either breast. In both breasts the lesions had an intraductile component. Distant metastasis was not evident. Bilateral radical mastectomy was performed and the patient was alive and well 6 years later.

Case 7. — A 54-year-old woman had a scirrhous adenocarcinoma, grade 4, directly under the nipple of the left breast without nodal involvement. An adenocarcinoma, grade 4, was present in the upper outer quadrant of the right breast without nodal involvement. The lesions in both breasts contained an intraductile component. Evidence of distant metastasis was not apparent on examination. The patient was alive and well, without evidence of recurrence or metastasis, when seen 1½ years after bilateral radical mastectomy. After this time she was lost to follow-up.

Case 8. — The left breast of a 73-year-old woman contained a medullary adenocarcinoma, grade 3, in the upper outer quadrant. The medial half of the right breast contained a mucinous adenocarcinoma, grade 2, just to the left of the nipple. Nodal involvement was not present in either axilla. There was no evidence of distant metastasis. The microscopic morphology of the two lesions is distinctly different. The patient was alive and well without evidence of recurrence or metastasis 3½ years after bilateral radical mastectomy.

It is of interest that of these eight patients only one (case 2) is presumed to have died of metastatic carcinoma. Of the remaining seven, one died of an unassociated disease, one was lost to follow-up after 1¹/₂ years, and five are known to be alive and well from 3¹/₂ to 8 years after bilateral radical mastectomy. This is in contrast to the gloomy prognosis usually accorded to patients having bilateral simultaneous breast cancers. This series is too small, however, to permit any general conclusions regarding the prognosis in all patients with bilateral independent simultaneous cancers of the breast. The fact should be reemphasized also that the criteria used to establish the lesions as probably independent simultaneous lesions were relatively rigid. If all patients with bilateral simultaneous involvement of the breasts were to be studied, the lesion in the second breast would undoubtedly be a metastatic lesion in a significant proportion, and the prognosis would be considerably less favorable, as indeed was the case in HARRINGTON's series.

e) Independent Cancers of the Second Breast in Association with Other Primary Malignant Neoplasms

Five, or 4.2 %, of the 118 patients who were proved to have primary cancers in both breasts had other, independent malignant neoplasms. Two of the five had carcinomas of the fundus uteri, two had carcinomas of the stomach, and one had generalized lymphosarcoma.

f) Comment

In mammary carcinoma, each breast represents the same tissue in the same person and is presumably exposed to the same carcinogenic influence, be it abnormal estrogenic stimulus or other factors as yet unrecognized. When carcinoma appears in one breast, the opposite breast must be assumed to have an increased vulnerability to the development of simultaneous or future malignant change.

Studies of KILGORE, MIDER and associates, HARRINGTON, and others have shown this thesis to be as true in fact as it seems in theory. The not infrequent occurrence of carcinoma in the second breast is well documented. It is the responsibility of the physician to be constantly aware of a potential malignant growth in the second breast.

g) The Problem of Prophylactic Simple Mastectomy of the Second Breast

It seems well established by this and other studies that the woman who has shown herself susceptible to mammary cancer because she has had a proved carcinoma of one breast runs a small but definite risk of a second carcinoma developing in the opposite breast. In the woman who survives her initial lesion, the rate of this risk probably ranges from 6 to 8 %. This conclusion must lead the physician to ask if removal of the opposite breast is justifiable in an attempt to provide the patient with a maximal chance of long-term survival. This departure from conventional management has its strong protagonists, of whom PACK has probably been the most outstanding. There are ,however, equally strong antagonists, most notably GUISS. He has proposed the existence of some immune factor against breast cancer and is of the opinion that the appearance of cancer in the second breast would "remobilize" this control mechanism; therefore, if prophylactic simple mastectomy were performed, "the patient's chances for long-term survival might be seriously curtailed rather than enhanced." Such a theory seems to have little foundation in fact, however, and KILGORE and associates have recently challenged the logic of this proposal.

Other authors including HUBBARD, SANDERS and GRIFFIN, KILGORE, and DOBSON, recommend prophylactic simple mastectomy for selected patients. Suggested criteria for selection have included a strong family history of cancer of the breast, premenopausal patients desiring future pregnancy, and patients with carcinoma, stage I. Contralateral mastectomy as a therapeutic as well as a prophylactic measure has been advocated for patients with lesions of the medial hemisphere because of the possibility of metastasis to the contralateral breast; considering the frequency of involvement of internal mammary lymph nodes in such cases, however, the advisability of therapeutic contralateral mastectomy without dissection of ipsilateral internal mammary nodes might be questioned.

The attitude of many physicians on this question is probably best expressed by YEATES: "Routine prophylactic (non-radical) removal of the opposite normal breast at the same time as radical mastectomy for the affected breast is theoretically sound and could become the accepted practice of the future. It is likely, however, that any surgeon in this country giving such a counsel would find himself without candidates." To compromise principle in this manner might be justifiable if, indeed, the objections of the patient were so strong. That the presupposed aversion of patients to this procedure may be exaggerated has been suggested by a recent trial series of DOBSON, who reported that 13 patients with carcinoma of the breast were offered prophylactic simple mastectomy by a simple statement of the facts without any effort to frighten the patient and without insistence on the procedure. Of the 13 patients, 11 accepted. Several months after operation all 11 patients stated that they were glad they had had it done.

Of still greater significance is the more recent experimental study at the University of Minnesota reported by HUBBARD. Contralateral prophylactic simple mastectomy was performed in conjunction with radical mastectomy on each of 16 patients whose diagnosis before operation was unilateral cancer of the breast. Two of the 16 patients were found to have clinically undetected small cancers in the breast that was removed prophylactically.

A seemingly reasonable approach to this problem was presented by KILGORE and associates, who proposed that the intelligent, well-balanced patient should be presented with the facts and permitted to decide whether one or both breasts should be removed. The emotionally stable patient would be frankly informed that even after successful treatment of cancer in a single breast a small but definite risk exists of a second cancer developing in the remaining breast. Prophylactic simple mastectomy should be performed if the patient chooses to have the benefit of this additional security. If the risk of retaining the opposite breast is elected, the patient should then be impressed with the need for frequent follow-up examinations and should be instructed carefully in the technique of self-examination.

Regardless of how compelling the arguments for prophylactic simple mastectomy might be, the fact remains that these arguments have been made for many years without convincing the rank and file of practicing surgeons. It is unlikely that the future will produce any change in their aversion to this procedure. Fortunately, however, it seems that the newly developed techniques of mammography may well obviate prophylactic simple mastectomy. BYRNE and associates have reported that of 102 patients examined by mammography after unilateral mastectomy for carcinoma, 6 have been found to have malignant lesions in the opposite breast. Five of these were unsuspected clinically. During a 2-year period MISSAKIAN and associates studied 397 such patients. Thorough physical examination plus mammography revealed carcinomas of the remaining breast in 25 patients, all of which were later confirmed pathologically. This represents an incidence to the date of their report of more than 6 %. Both of these studies have been performed over relatively short periods of time, and yet a striking incidence of bilateral breast cancers has already been reported. As they progress it seems quite likely that HARRINGTON's estimate of a 6 to 8 % incidence of bilateral breast cancers may prove to be less than the true incidence. The value of mammography in detecting carcinoma in the remaining breast seems well established. If prophylactic simple mastectomy is not to be performed, there is no alternative to the inclusion of mammography in the thoughtful treatment of the woman with breast carcinoma. It would seem ill advised for any surgeon to undertake the treatment of a breast carcinoma unless he is also prepared to offer and advise the protection of skillfully interpreted mammography performed before initial surgery and periodically thereafter.

Summary

Practical and objective criteria have been presented for the diagnosis of independent cancer in the second breast.

At the Mayo Clinic 118 cases were found in which the established criteria were recognized during a 10-year period. These cases represent an overall known incidence of independent cancer of the second breast of 4.0 % (3.7 % unsimultaneous cancers, 0.27 % simultaneous cancers).

It must be emphasized that these figures represent only the known rate of occurrence and are calculated on the basis of all breast cancer patients. The true incidence among those patients surviving their initial breast cancer would be considerably higher.

From a theoretical standpoint, the frequency of development of cancer in the second breast is not surprising, since carcinogenic factors which have induced malignant change in one breast may also be expected to exert a similar influence on the remaining mammary tissue.

The cumulative evidence in this study and in the literature indicates that prophylactic simple mastectomy of the second breast in patients treated for unilateral breast cancer may be an effective and a patient-acceptable means of increasing the long-term survival in patients with mammary cancer. This procedure, however, has not been accepted by the practicing surgeon and does seem likely to become accepted. A reasonable and, indeed, almost mandatory alternative is mammography of the opposite breast performed before surgery and periodically after surgery. This should, of course, supplement frequent follow-up examinations and careful intruction of the patient in the technique of self-examination.

As an essential part of the management of breast carcinoma, the physician must be constantly alert to the potential malignant change in the second breast.

References

BYRNE, R. N., L. S. BRINGHURST, and J. GERSHON-COHEN: Postoperative detection of cancer by periodic mammography of remaining breast. Surg. Gynec. Obstet. 115, 282 (1962).

CARROLL, W. W., and T. W. SHIELDS: Bilateral simultaneous breast cancer. Arch. Surg. 70, 672 (1955).

DOBSON, LEONARD: The problem of bilateral nonsimultaneous breast cancer. Stanf. med. Bull. 13, 456 (1955).

GUISS, L. W.: The problem of bilateral independent mammary carcinoma. Amer. J. Surg. 88, 171 (1954).

HARRINGTON, S. W.: Survival rates of radical mastectomy for unilateral and bilateral carcinoma of the breast. Surgery 19, 154 (1946).

HUBBARD, T. B., JR.: Nonsimultaneous bilateral carcinoma of the breast. Surgery 34, 706 (1953).

KILGORE, A. R.: The incidence of cancer in the second breast after radical removal of one breast for cancer. J. Amer. med. Ass. 77, 454, (1921).

—, H. G. BELL, and R. E. AHLQUIST, JR.: Cancer in the second breast. Amer. J. Surg. 92, 156 (1956).

MIDER, G. B., J. A. SCHILLING, J. C. DONOVAN, and E. S. RENDALL: Multiple cancer: A study of other cancers arising in patients with primary malignant neoplasms of the stomach, uterus, breast, large intestine, or hematopoietic system. Cancer (Philad.) 5, 1104 (1952).

MISSAKIAN, M. M., D. M. WITTEN, and E. G. HARRISON, JR.: Mammography after mastectomy: Usefulness in search for recurrent carcinoma of breast. J. Amer. med. Ass. 191, 1045 (1965).

NISBET, WILLIAM: A case of the cure of cancer of both breasts, the one ulcerated, the other scirrhous. Med. Phys. J. 4, 296 (1800).

PACK, G. T.: Argument for bilateral mastectomy. (Editorial.) Surgery 29, 929 (1951).

PIERCE, E. H., J. W. KIRKLIN, J. R. McDONALD, and R. P. GAGE: Carcinoma in the medial and lateral halves of the breast. Surg. Gynec. Obstet. 103, 759 (1956).

SANDERS, G. B., and D. W. GRIFFIN: Bilatral mastectomy for breast cancer. Sth. med. J. (Bgham, Ala.) 46, 1083 (1953).

YEATES, J. M.: Bilateral carcinoma of the breast. Med. J. Aust. 2, 54 (1953).

12. Bilateral Testicular Cancers

On the 6th of June 1795 (the day after the Cirencester East-Indiaman sailed from Portsmouth), James Foster, aetat. 35, who had the preceding night succeeded in imposing himself on the ship as a healthy seaman, was discovered to be entirely unfit for duty, in consequence of cancer affecting both testicles and spermatic cords. (LIVINGSTONE, 1805.)

A hundred and fifty years after this report, ABESHOUSE and associates were able to collect a total of 209 cases of bilateral malignant neoplasms of the testes from the literature. Although this total may be relatively small, the incidence of bilateral lesions among patients with testicular cancer is striking. In a statistical study HAMILTON and GILBERT reported the general incidence of malignant tumors of the testis to be 0.0013 %. In a review of 7,000 cases of malignant tumors of the testis, they found 144 (2.1 %) to be bilateral. They stated that in men with one testicular cancer the likelihood of cancer in the second testis is from several hundred to several thousand times greater than that expected in chance association. They also found that the incidence of involvement of the second testis rose sharply when both testes were ectopic; it was 15 % in cases of inguinal cryptorchism and 30 % in cases of abdominal cryptorchism.

The question may be raised of the possibility that the lesion in the second testis may be metastatic or result from local spread from the initial lesion. Most of the articles in the literature, however, seem to be in agreement with ABESHOUSE and associates, who stated that the occasional occurrence of tumors of different histologic types as well as the absence of demonstrable vascular or lymphatic communications between the two testes strongly favors the concept that both testicular tumors are primary. The pointed out also that metastatic tumors to the testes from other sites are extremely rare and that not a single case of bilateral chorioepithelioma has been reported despite the fact that this tumor freqently is reponsible for widespread metastasis.

During the 10-year period of this study, a total of 226 patients who had pathologically confirmed malignant tumors of the testis (exclusive of lymphomas) were seen at the Mayo Clinic. Of this group, five (2.2%) had bilateral cancers. Four of these patients had simultaneous bilateral seminomas, and one had a seminoma and a teratocarcinoma that did not occur simultaneously.

The clinical importance of this problem has been emphasized by HARPER and associates who said: "The danger is so great that any patient who has a testicular cancer requires close and indefinite continued observation of the remaining gonad.... Prophylactic orchidectomy is suggested when the remaining testis is sterile and presents a cancer risk."

References

ABESHOUSE, B. S., ANTONIO TIONGSON, and MORTON GOLDFARB: Bilateral tumors of testicles: Review of literature and report of case of bilateral simultaneous lymphosarcoma. J. Urol. (Baltimore) 74, 522 (1955).

HAMILTON, J. B., and J. B. GILBERT: Studies in malignant tumors of the testis. IV. Bilateral testicular cancer: Incidence, nature, and bearing upon management of the patient with a single testicular cancer. Cancer Res. 2, 125 (1942).

HARPER, J. G. M., S. B. DEWING, and G. NAGAMATSU: Bilateral carcinoma of testis: Report of 3 cases. J. Urol. (Baltimore) 71, 634 (1954).

LIVINGSTONE, JOHN: A case of cancer of both testicles, which terminated favourably by the supervention of scurvy. Edinb. med. surg. J. 1, 163 (1805).

13. Bilateral Ovarian Carcinomas

Bilateral ovarian carcinoma is exceedingly common. In a review of several series of cases in the literature, GEIST found that the reported incidence of bilateral lesions varied from 21.5 to 90.9%. DOCKERTY and MASSON stated that bilateral lesions are found on gross inspection in about 40% of cases of ovarian cystadenocarcinomas, whereas microscopic examination will reveal them in considerably more than 50%. These authors also estimated that 50% of solid ovarian cancers are found to involve both gonads.

In contrast to the male gonad, the ovary is frequently the site of metastatic carcinoma, especially in cases of carcinomas of the pelvic organs. Although bilateral ovarian cancers often may arise as two independent primary lesions, it was impossible with the criteria and methods of our study to distinguish such a case with certainty from a single primary lesion with metastasis to the contralateral ovary.

Only one case of bilateral ovarian carcinoma was felt to be acceptable to the present study, that of a woman who had a resection for carcinoma of the right ovary at the age of 28 years. Seven years later she returned with an encapsulated low-grade cystadenocarcinoma of the left ovary and no evidence of metastasis.

Regardless of whether bilateral ovarian cancers are multicentric malignant neoplasms or metastatic lesions from a single malignant focus, the frequency of bilateral lesions cannot be ignored in the management of the patient with malignant disease of an ovary. DOCKERTY and MASSON's conclusion should be reemphasized. They said that as a general rule panhysterectomy should be advised for all ovarian carcinomas, even if one ovary is normal on gross inspection.

References

DOCKERTY, M. B., and J. C. MASSON: Clinical features, types and grades of malignant ovarian tumors. Surg. Clin. N. Amer. *Aug.*, 1201 (1941).

GEIST, S. H.: Ovarian tumors. New York: Paul B. Hoeber, Inc. 1944, pp. 120—121.

14. Multicentric Bronchial Carcinomas

Multiple pulmonary carcinomas were not included in this study, because of the problem encountered in establishing beyond reasonable doubt that these lesions are not metastatic from a single neoplastic focus. SHIELDS and associates in 1964 collected 53 cases of grossly recognizable bilateral bronchogenic carcinoma from the literature and added 3 of their own; they freely admitted the difficulty of authenticating many of these cases. There would seem to be little doubt, however, that many, if not all, bronchogenic carcinomas present with multiple areas of in situ carcinoma at some stage in their development. Three studies presented in 1952 (BLACK and ACKERMAN; McGRATH and associates, and WILLIAMS) documented the microscopic multicentricity of bronchial cancer. The frequency of occurrence of this phenomenon was demonstrated by AUERBACH and co-workers when they showed either borderline or definite carcinoma in situ in 48 of 54 cases of bronchial carcinoma. In five cases these areas showed evidence of early invasion. RYAN and McDONALD studied autopsy specimens of the opposite lung in 39 patients who had previously undergone pneumonectomy for bronchogenic carcinoma. Five of these 39 patients showed definite areas of in situ carcinoma in the remaining lung. Throughout these studies smoking has been emphasized as strongly associated with the observations of squamous metaplasia and in situ carcinomatous change. The imposing frequency of multicentric carcinomatous change undoubtedly plays a role in the overall poor surgical results in bronchogenic carcinoma. The great importance of prohibiting further use of tobacco following surgical treatment of lung cancer must be emphasized.

References

AUERBACH, OSCAR, J. B. GERE, J. M. PAWLOWSKI, G. E. MEUHSAM, H. J. SMOLIN, and A. P. STOUT: Carcinoma-in-situ and early invasive carcinoma occurring in the tracheobronchial trees in cases of bronchial carcinoma. J. thorac. Surg. 34, 298 (1957).

BLACK, HARRISON, and L. V. ACKERMAN: The importance of epidermoid carcinoma *in situ* in the histogenesis of carcinoma of the lung. Ann. Surg. 136, 44 (1952).

McGRATH, E. J., E. A. GALL, and D. P. KESSLER: Bronchogenic carcinoma, a product of multiple sites of origin. J. thorac. Surg. 24, 271 (1952).

RYAN, R. F., and J. R. McDONALD: Bronchogenic carcinoma with in situ carcinoma in the opposite lung: Report of five cases. Proc. Mayo Clin. 31, 478 (1956).

SHIELDS, T. W., C. T. DRAKE, and J. C. SHERRICK: Bilateral primary bronchogenic carcinoma. J. thorac. Surg. 48, 401 (1964).

WILLIAMS, MARJORIE J.: Extensive carcinoma in situ in the bronchial mucosa associated with two invasive bronchogenic carcinomas: Report of case. Cancer (Philad.) 5, 740 (1952).

15. Multicentric Carcinomas of Parenchymatous Organs

a) Multicentric Carcinomas of the Kidney

Unilateral multicentric renal carcinomas of the hypernephroma type are not uncommon. Of the 487 cases of hypernephroma proved at the Mayo Clinic during the period covered by this study, a total of 22 cases (4.5%) showed two or more discrete tumors within the same kidney. Here again, we were confronted by the problem of distinguishing true multicentric lesions from local metastatic lesions from a single primary focus. On careful study of the gross and microscopic changes in these cases, we accepted only 4 of the 22 cases as representing multiple primary lesions beyond any reasonable doubt and therefore acceptable to the criteria of this study.

Although bilateral Wilms' tumors are not unusual, bilateral hypernephromas are rare. In 1955, HERMANN and LIEBERMAN could collect only 25 cases from the world literature. Only three cases could be found in the present study, and in each of these, one of the two lesions was an incidental finding at autopsy.

b) Multicentric Carcinomas of the Thyroid and Pancreas

Multiple discrete areas of carcinoma of the thyroid or pancreas are observed occasionally. In some of these cases the lesions may represent true multicentric neoplasms, but the possibility of local metastasis via lymphatic or vascular channels from a single malignant focus cannot be ruled out in the individual case. Cases of multiple carcinomatous lesions of the thyroid or pancreas, therefore, were not included in the present study.

c) Multicentric Hepatomas

Probably a majority of patients who have hepatomas in cirrhotic livers have multiple hepatomas when they are first present clinically. Of 10 cases in which hepatomas were seen at autopsy at this clinic during the period under this study, 6 (60%) were found to have two or more carcinomatous foci. Here again it would be impossible to state with any certainty that these lesions are true multicentric cancers rather than local metastatic lesions from a single primary cancer. These cases were not included in the present study.

Reference

HERMANN, H. B., and M. L. LIEBERMAN: Bilateral renal carcinoma. N. Y. med. J. **55**, 1915 (1955).

16. Multicentric Gliomas of the Central Nervous System

Multicentricity in cerebral gliomas has been a subject of considerable interest ever since the initial case was reported by VIRCHOW in 1864. Although opinions differ about the possibility of multiple lesions representing local metastasis from a single focus of glioma, the bulk of the literature is in agreement with the statement of COURVILLE, who said: "For the most part the occurrence of multiple gliomas is to be explained on the basis of development of multiple primary foci."

SCHERER stated that about 10% of all gliomas are primary multicentric growths, half of which are macroscopically visible as multiple tumors. In 1936 COURVILLE collected 134 cases from the world literature, including those which he reported. In his own series he found multiple lesions in 21 of 269 cases of glioma (7.8%).

In 1963, by reviewing the literature, BATZDORF and MALAMUD found nine major studies of gliomas in which the frequency of multicentricity was recorded. The incidence of this phenomenon ranged from 0.9 to 10.0%. In their own study they found that 5 of 209 patients (2.4%) with gliomas had multicentric lesions.

Cases included in our series are derived entirely from routine neuropathologic examination at autopsy. Fifteen multiple gliomas were found among a total of 305 cases of glioma proved at autopsy during the period under study. This represents an overall incidence of 4.9%. It is of interest that these occurred in 5 of 196 males (2.6%) and in 10 of the 109 females (9.2%). Twelve were cases of multiple astrocytomas, one of multiple ependymomas, one of astrocytoma plus an oligodendroglioma, and one of an astrocytoma plus multiple ependymomas. In 13 cases, all lesions were confined to the brain; in 1 case there was a lesion in the spinal cord as well as lesions in the brain; and in 1 case a high-grade astrocytoma involved the cerebral cortex and a small low-grade astrocytoma involved the neurohypophysis.

References

BATZDORF, ULRICH, and NATHAN MALAMUD: The problem of multicentric gliomas. J. Neurosurg. 20, 122 (1963).

COURVILLE, C. B.: Multiple primary tumors of the brain: Review of the literature and report of twenty-one cases. Amer. J. Cancer. 26, 703 (1936).

SCHERER, J. H.: Critical review: Pathology of cerebral gliomas. J. Neurol. Psychiat. 3, 147 (1940).

VIRCHOW: Cited by COURVILLE, C. B.

17. Multicentric Malignant Neoplasms of the Reticuloendothelial System

SLAUGHTER as well as others have suggested that the malignant diseases of the reticuloendothelial system — that is, leukemia, lymphoma, multiple myeloma, and Kaposi's sarcoma — may represent extreme examples of the multicentricity of origin of malignant neoplasms. Certainly lymphomas, multiple myeloma, or Kaposi's sarcoma often may involve widely separated focal areas in the earlier stages of the disease and later may show more generalized dissemination. Our present knowledge of the nature and pathogenesis of these disease processes is so scant, however, that it is premature to conclude that they should be classified with the other examples of multicentric malignant neoplasms discussed in this presentation.

Reference

SLAUGHTER, D. P.: The multiplicity of origin of malignant tumors: Collective review. Int. Abstr. Surg. 79, 89 (1944).

18. The Case for Multicentricity of Origin of Malignant Neoplasms

The present concept of the multicentric origin of malignant neoplasms is perhaps best expressed in the words of WILLIS (1945), who said:

In human as in experimental carcinogenesis the effective stimuli are applied, not to one cell or one small group of cells, but to a more or less extensive area of epithelial tissue. All the epithelium in that area is acted upon similarly, though of course usually not equally. Neoplasia will commence where stimuli have been maximal, but the neoplastic response will later be manifested by neighboring tissue that was subjected to the same original stimuli.

To expand on this thesis, our present knowledge of oncology has tended to show that carcinogenesis is not an isolated biologic accident. It rather seems to be the result of specific intrinsic or extrinsic carcinogenic influences acting on a susceptible tissue for a sufficient time to initiate irreversible anaplastic change in the reproductive pattern of the constituent cells. Carcinoma in its broadest sense then is not a unicellular disease but a disease of an entire tissue or a large portion of it.

Before the development of frank anaplasia the tissue sometimes seems to be in a premalignant state. In some tissues this may be evidenced by grossly visible hyperplastic premalignant lesions such as leukoplakia or the adenomatous polyp. A variable time later, multiple areas of in situ carcinomatous change will begin at the point of maximal carcinogenic stimulus. The areas of in situ carcinomatous change may coalesce into a single carcinoma, or they may form two or more discrete multicentric carcinomas. This chain of events is depicted diagrammatically in Fig. 18. By careful and detailed histologic studies these relationships have been demonstrated in carcinoma of the skin by WILLIS (1944 and 1945) and by MOLESWORTH, in carcinoma of the lip by WARWICK, in carcinoma of the oral cavity by SLAUGHTER, in gastric carcinoma by COLLINS and GALL, in carcinoma of the cervix by CARSON and GALL, in carcinoma of the breast by QUALHEIM and GALL, and in bronchogenic carcinoma by a number of investigators.

Carrying this thesis one step further, SLAUGHTER suggested that many so-called local recurrences may be new foci of cancer arising in the peripheral field of a previously treated cancer. Tumors may form at the site of a previously treated cancer in three ways as follows: (1) A true recurrence may result either from incomplete removal of the initial lesion or from implantation of tumor cells during the surgical procedure. (2) A second cancer may develop from an unrecognized in situ carcinoma present at the time of the initial resection. (3) A second cancer may develop in the adjacent tissue which was rendered precancerous by the same stimuli which incited the initial neoplasm. These mechanisms are described diagrammatically in Fig. 19.

In support of the concept that a significant number of supposed local recurrences are in fact new tumors, LONG and associates presented a careful histologic study of 31 lesions previously diagnosed as recurrent carcinomas of the colon occurring at the site of anastomosis. They found a transitional zone of progressive anaplastic change between the normal bowel mucosa and the main carcinoma in nine of these lesions. They concluded that this transition zone established the second lesions as new and independent growths.

The concept that carcinoma is frequently a multicentric disease is well supported. The rates of occurrence of clinically significant multicentric cancer in this and other studies show that it is a common problem. The fact that carcinoma is often multicentric must be considered in the thoughtful management of the patient with malignant disease if maximal long-term survival is to be obtained. If a tissue is the site of a carcinoma, the entire tissue should be removed if this can be done without undue risk, functional impairment, or cosmetic deformity. If this cannot be done, the remaining tissue should be observed frequently and carefully for an indefinite period for the possible development of a new growth. All lesions known or suspected to be premalignant should be eradicated promptly after their discovery. The attack against the recurrent lesion must be equally as vigorous as that launched against the initial

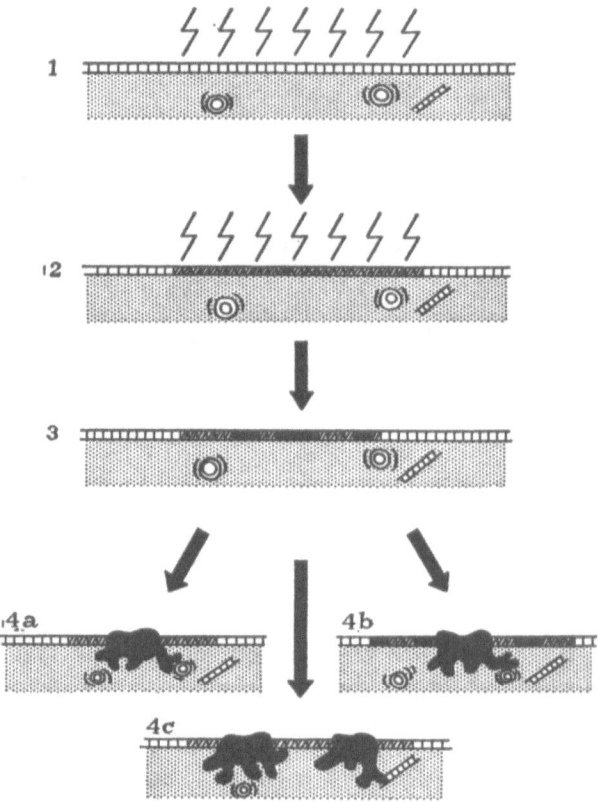

Fig 18. Mechanisms of single and multicentric carcinoma formation. 1, Susceptible tissue exposed to carcinogenic stimuli. 2, Tissue in a premalignant state exposed to continued carcinogenic stimuli. 3, In situ carcinomatous change. 4a, Single carcinoma. 4b, Single carcinoma with multicentric areas of in situ carcinomatous change. 4c, Multicentric invasive carcinomas

neoplasm. The physician who assumes the responsibility of treating the patient with carcinoma must assume also the responsibility of constant vigilance to detect and promptly treat the multicentric lesions to which they may be prone.

References

CARSON, R. P., and E. A. GALL: Preinvasive carcinoma and precancerous metaplasia of the cervix: A serial block survey. Amer. J. Path. 30, 15 (1954).

COLLINS, W. T., and E. A. GALL: Gastric carcinoma: A multicentric lesion. Cancer (Philad.) 5, 62 (1952).

LONG, J. W., C. W. MAYO, M. B. DOCKERTY, and E. S. JUDD, JR.: Recurrent versus new and independent carcinomas of the colon and rectum. Proc. Mayo Clin. 25, 169 (1950).

MOLESWORTH, E. H.: Rodent ulcer. Med. J. Aust. 1, 878 (1927).

QUALHEIM, R. E., and E. A. GALL: Breast carcinoma with multiple sites of origin. Cancer (Philad.) 10, 460 (1957).

SLAUGHTER, D. P.: Multicentric origin of intraoral carcinoma. Surgery. 20, 133 (1946).

WARWICK, MARGARET: Model of carcinoma of the lip reconstructed from serial section. J. Amer. med. Ass. 82, 1119 (1924).

WILLIS, R. A.: The mode of origin of tumors: Solitary localized squamous cell growths of the skin. Cancer Res. 4, 630 (1944).

— Further studies on the mode of origin of carcinomas of the skin. Cancer Res. 5, 469 (1945).

Summary

This study has shown that the incidence of grossly recognizable multicentric epithelial cancers is substantial. In studies by other authors the incidence of microscopic multicentricity in epithelial cancers has ranged from 22 to as high as 93 %. Also it has been demonstrated that just as epithelial malignant disease is not always spatially unicentric, likewise it is not always temporally unicentric, for a large percentage of the multicentric cancers have appeared months or years after excision of an initial lesion.

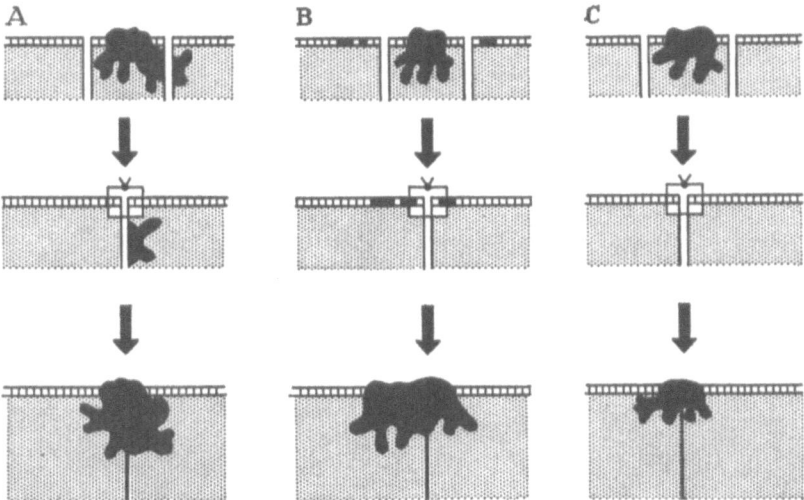

Fig. 19. Mechanisms of tumor formation at the site of excision of a malignant neoplasm. A, True recurrence arising from tumor cells either implanted or unexcised at the time of surgery. B, Second lesion arising from neighboring in situ carcinoma present at the time of surgery. C, Second lesion developing in adjacent tissue which was normal at the time of surgery but which had been subjected to the same carcinogenic stimuli which incited the initial lesion

In light of these observations, the traditional concept of carcinoma as a single neoplasm intruding in an otherwise normal tissue is not tenable. In a significant number of cases, the initial neoplasm is only the first and most obvious manifestation of a carcinogenic disease process that may involve a large portion or all of a given tissue. Further evolution of this carcinogenic process in the surrounding tissue may contribute to the local extension of the initial lesion, or it may produce multicentric lesions at varying periods after the initial lesion. If the entire initial lesion has been removed surgically, progression of the carcinogenic process in the adjacent tissue may produce new lesions at or near the site of excision that may be grossly indistinguishable from true recurrence.

Recognition of the multicentric origin of malignant disease should play a significant role in the tactics employed by the physician when he joins the patient in the life or death struggle against a malignant neoplasm. Carcinoma frequently may be a disease of an entire tissue or a large segment thereof rather than a single neoplasm. In surgical treatment, therefore, it seems rational to excise the entire tissue if this can be accomplished without disabling functional or cosmetic impairment and without prohibitive surgical risk. If this cannot be done, then the physician must impress on the patient the importance of frequent and regular follow-up examinations. Pre-malignant lesions must be eradicated promptly, and, in the absence of distant metastasis, the "recurrence" must be treated with the same vigor as the initial lesion.

Herstellung: Konrad Triltsch, Graphischer Betrieb, Würzburg